The choice is yours and always has been

Why Not Stay Fat?

All your questions answered

Wayne Lambert

WHY NOT STAY FAT?

By Wayne Lambert

Certified Personal Trainer, Nutrition Specialist and Master Life Coach

C.E.O & Founder – Whole Body Workshop and Weight Loss Dubai

Author of Psychology of weight loss, Visualise the new you, Exercise your whole body at home, Maximise your fitness potential and Exercise Therapy - rehab exercises.

ISBN 978-0-9561494-3-5

I dedicate this book to my wife Laila, who all her life has helped so many people with their health and well being through holistic healing and life coaching.

Laila is one in a million and second to noone, she is a gentle and spiritual soul who continues to inspire me everyday with her unselfish plight in giving to others.

May this book provide you with everything you desire.

TABLE OF CONTENTS

PREFACE

This is now my 6th and final book which relates directly as to what I set out to do 2 years ago, which was to put pen to paper and share my knowledge with the world. Prior to this decision though, it took me some time to understand that education and learning is an ongoing process and should never really end, so the best thing for me to do was to start writing and see where it led to. Consequently I still managed to continue with certain educational courses alongside writing, which obviously tested me somewhat.

My health & fitness career spans across almost 2 decades now, with my qualifications in this chosen field being current and regularly updated. Writing books, creating fitness DVDs and audio books about health, fitness and in particular weight loss, gives me a tremendous sense of achievement. My special interest in weight loss can be put down to my studies in nutrition and my experiences with personal training, but it was within my research in psychology that has helped me understand about the bigger picture and how we must take into account the mind and body concept as a whole, hence naming the company Whole Body Workshop.

Since meeting my wife Laila I have learned so much, mostly about how we as humans operate, and how our own thoughts contribute immensely to what holds us back the most in life. You don't have to be religious or spiritual to believe in a higher being, but it certainly helps to understand that if we think bad thoughts about ourselves or others, then this is what we will ultimately attract. I do not cover religion, beliefs or spirituality in this book, but you will read for yourself that what we want to achieve in this lifetime, is as much about our minds as it is our bodies, and we need to develop them both, not one or the other.

I believe that we must do as much as we can within each given day, so that when we lie in bed at night at least we can say that we have done everything we possibly can. Most people honestly believe that they have no time for the important things in life, and tend to take their bodies for granted. The importance of a healthy body is something many individuals will quite possibly never truly understand until of course it is too late.

The fact that you are reading this book is obviously due to your self awareness or even curiosity as to finding out what the answers are. The fact is, the answers remain within each of us, we have the solutions and we have all the tools and resources within our mind and body to move forwards, deleting past attempts and renewing our thought processes with positive actions. Only then will we realise that our own life purpose is quite simply to respect our bodies. The human body is only capable of carrying us forward so far, and then one day it will just give up without too much warning.

The idea of this book is to educate the reader about the global health issues related to the constant abuse of the human body, so that each family can go about their life listening to their bodies, preferably before the warning signs come and it's too late.

THE MOST COMMON FREQUENTLY ASKED QUESTIONS

"It's not what you know; it's what you learn after you know it that counts."

- John Wooden

Why do people fail at weight loss and what are the risks?

Conventional diets just don't work. Approximately five out of six people who try to lose weight fail, and a very high percentage of those who do succeed in losing weight gain all the weight back within two years. If you drop your calories and go hungry, forcing your body to lose weight, your body will fight back. This is your bodies built in "intelligence." It reacts as if you are starving your body and will do everything it can to preserve your fat. When you lose weight by starving yourself, you lose important muscle, bone, fluids, and even vital organ mass. What is not widely known is that the risk of health problems starts when someone is only very slightly overweight, and that the likelihood of problems increases as someone becomes more and more overweight. Many of these conditions cause long term suffering for individuals and families. In addition, the costs for the health care system can be extremely high. What people need to ask themselves is "how long did it take me to put this weight on?" And the answer is more than likely going to be "over a long period of time." The difference being that most people don't even notice the weight "creeping" up before it's actually too late and when it comes to losing it, they all of a sudden expect to actually see it disappearing before their very eyes and because they don't, they give up because it's taking too long.

Whatever attempts people have tried in the past to lose weight, they have either been lied to or they have demanded too much weight loss too soon and, therefore, the expectations have been set far too high. The time that it took to put on weight would ultimately have depended on how active that person was during that period of weight gain and the probability would be that they were quite active at a younger age, therefore it would have taken a long time to put it on and, unfortunately, they are now more than likely living an inactive lifestyle. In short, your body is too smart for short-term quick fixes to ever work because your body will always fight back to maintain a natural balance or, as it is called, "homeostasis." For every crash diet you go on or diet pill you take, there will always be an equal or greater valley or low point, which basically means that if you over stimulate, your body can respond by slowing down your natural metabolic rate (i.e. your body's fat burners) to compensate. As a result, when you stop the diet or using the stimulant, your metabolism is slower than ever and you gain back any weight you lost and more. Those people with what we call "quick fix disease" want to take a pill, go to sleep and wake up skinny. These people are forever on a quest to bypass hard work and find short cuts to health and fitness goals that normally take months or years to attain.

What is the correct way to lose weight?

It's important to choose a diet plan that is effective and comfortable. Ideally, it should be a plan that can be sustained over a long period of time, and it should allow you the liberty to eat out at restaurants every once in a while. Try to deal with the issues related to food that you might have, such as, emotional eating, binging, purging, obsessing, anorexia or even a drug addiction. Figure out if you're actually trying to hide your emotional issues behind your extra weight. You can only tackle the problem by attacking its root. You can only get to the root of the problem by considering issues like eating disorders, body image problems, and fear of intimacy, emotional issues or food addiction, which you might have. You have to know why you're overweight to be able to solve the problem. You can then proceed to live your life comfortably and with confidence. Once called fat farms, adult weight loss camps may provide the correct motivation to lose weight, and keep it off for good. A good adult weight loss camp should be about more than restricting diets and a strict workout plan. It would be most beneficial if it provides you with a spiritual outlook and experience, and on the whole they should improve your health, lifestyle, body image, and intellectual issues. You should also be instructed on how hunger works, so that you may address it once you return home. It should also teach you the difference between weight loss supplements and diet pills. Dieting usually isn't very successful because it often requires you to eat specific foods in a certain combination, and such a method cannot be sustained over a long period of time. Long term weight loss would entail changing your habits for several decades at least. When starting on a new diet you have to ask yourself if you can sustain it even when you're old. If you have a family to feed, then find out if they'll be comfortable following the new menu, or if you'll be able to stay away from the pizzas and burgers they may choose to have. You can't be successful if you simply count your calories or weigh your food.

How will weight loss affect me as a person?

Weight Loss Psychology can help you to overcome many mental obstacles that are keeping you overweight. The general approach to losing weight is quite simply to reduce the number of calories you eat and increase the number of calories you burn by exercising. Its that simple. Most of us have all the reasons in the world to change something about ourselves but inevitably never seem to get round to it and therefore we are consistently 'almost' getting in shape. For a number of reasons we spend our life getting on and off the weight loss merry-go-round, wasting time, starting, stopping, and lying about our behaviour which includes making excuses and forever waiting for that right time to start (which never comes), getting frustrated, complaining about our genetics and generally being miserable. Creating physiological change whether it is to get bigger, smaller, faster, fitter, lighter or leaner seems to be more about our head than it is about our body. The weight loss process isn't as much about dumbbells, treadmills and carbohydrates as it is about attitude, thinking, beliefs, passion, self-control, decisions, standards and habits. Whole body workshop was named as such so that we could endeavour to provide anything whatsoever relevant to the body and mind. Everyday people want everyday solutions. Primarily, the website and the products within it are related to weight loss but with a continued effort we can assist those that need that extra push, whether it is with the mind or the body. We believe that psychology of weight loss is extremely important because it provides a foundation from which you can work from, very similar to the lifestyle challenges within 'Visualise The New You' book. Practically anyone can lose weight but those who manage to keep it off are a rare breed. Theirs is not an entirely mysterious phenomenon, they stay slim by maintaining the behaviours that got them there in the first place. They eat healthier foods, decrease portion sizes and exercise. But how, exactly, do they keep it up? The answer suggests a psychological overhaul as much as a physical one.

Make success a habit, You'll be surprised at what it makes you

What are the main things missing in weight loss programs?

It is difficult to control hunger pangs and starve one-self, also getting back to normal food has a yo-yo effect with one's weight. The reasons why a person grows obese is quite vague. There are books that say that fat people eat excessively out of a habit but this reference overlooks the psychological and emotional reasons. Again counsellors who write on this subject concentrate on the psychological problem only.

Here are four situations which say that excess fat is due to some psychological disorder:

1. Ponder over time when you had become slightly trim and had attained, even though not completely, your aim to shed those excess fat deposits. Think whether you had been extremely agile then or whether you were working out too often. In case your answer is yes then your fat had to do with some mental discomfort;

2. In case, after your past dieting attempts, you have put on more than a pound of fat in one week, it is most likely that your excess weight, before your dietary measure, was due to some mental crisis;

3. Bulimia and anorexia, the diseases associated with food problems, are in most cases due to some psychological problem;

4. Again your fat could be due to improper mental composure in case your devouring of foodstuff is sparked off by anxiety. You can take into account your mental and emotional difficulties, especially if you have started gaining weight during your teenage years. Probably they are the reasons why you cannot shed your excess fat. In case your excess weight is due to some intense emotional shock that you have confronted in those years, then you will have a tough time trying to become thin.

A very small number of people all over the world are successful in recognising the emotional problem that causes their abnormal fatness and immediately transform the problems into ways of being slim. However, most people confront many difficulties and undertake rigorous practices to become thin. They try all means possible knowing full well that in spite of all their efforts their being slim is not a result they can be sure of. Quite a number of books define emotionally stressing situations that give rise to the binging habit, however you may or may not benefit from them. Generally it is the emotional upheavals aswell as the various circumstances that we confront in life that increase our problems. Thus in order to escape from them, a person might endeavour to eat too much. If that makes him/her comfortable and stops fretting, then he/she continues to gorge. At times we run away from feelings such as love, annoyance, desire, sorrow etc and tend to find an alternative. We sometimes cannot come to terms with the idea that we are just another one in the rat race or maybe even certain factors about our sexual nature seems too hard to cope with.

At times people have parents who keep feeding their children or parents rebuke them by telling them that they will not be allowed to eat or any other such childhood shock related to food give rise to this problem. We always tend to consciously ignore that aspect about us which leaves us strained and weary because the moment any incident reminds us of that shock we are left drained psychologically. People who suffer from emotional distresses connected to food, then binge, the only remedy is to stay calm in such circumstances. However the person suffering from it will know that it is rather difficult. It requires a lot of willpower, strength aswell as pledge to relax in such situation and then gradually transform oneself. Looking upon fat as a sort of sign such as fear, a pain in the head or even an excess intake of alcohol helps to combat the problem. The emotional reasons that lead to these disorders are quite similar. The upcoming content of this book will assist you immensely in case you have recognised that the causes for your excess weight are emotional to a certain extent.

What available weight loss options are there?

Meal replacements
These are usually in the form of milkshakes, biscuits, snack bars and even chocolate and they are potentially extremely dangerous. Apart from doing nothing to encourage healthier, long term eating habits, they may not provide all the nutrients you require and could therefore lead to malnutrition and excessive weight loss.

Ready meals
In May of 1992, Food magazine analysed popular calorie-counted ready meals promoted as slimming aids. They found that they were all lacking in fibre and healthy fats.

Surgery
An increasingly large number of people are turning to surgery with an attitude of "If all else fails, cut it off or suck it out." Liposuction, perhaps the most common surgery, quite literally sucks out fat from under the skin and has seen a number of cases of post operative pain, infection and disfigurement. The fat sometimes grows back in lumps and middle aged and older people may be left with flabby, sagging skin. There is also the additional risk of blood clots, permanent numbness in the area, severe bruising, loss of blood and lowered immunity to infection. Besides, it can't be good to suck out fat from inside the stomach without the risk of damaging internal organs. Bypass surgery or gastric banding limits the amount of food you can take in and some operations also restrict the amount of food you can digest. Many people have this type of surgery to lose weight quickly but, if you follow diet and exercise recommendations, you can keep the majority of the weight off. The surgery option as explained has risks and complications, including infections, hernias and blood clots.

Diet plan only
Permanent or temporary weight loss, which will your new diet achieve? It's often easier, for short term results, to make drastic changes to your diet, although it seems to be

counterintuitive because starting a whole new eating plan tends to make things simple in the early days of a diet. You might hate the food and feel hungry but you know exactly what you can and can't eat and, if you follow the diet, you'll lose weight, simple as that. No decisions, no choices, no room for mistakes. Why then would I persuade people not to do that?

The reason is in the length of time such a solution lasts because most people have given up a drastic plan like this within a week or two, especially in January with New Year's resolutions. Either they can't get the ingredients one day, they hate the food, they were too hungry, they had a night out and couldn't eat according to the plan or quite simply went completely off the rails. Even if you manage to stick to the plan, what happens at the end of it after you lose weight? The problem is you have learned nothing new, you are right back where you were with your old habits and eating just as much as you always did. The weight comes right back as mentioned before, the classic yo-yo situation.

The way to achieve permanent weight loss is to make permanent adjustments to your diet and habits, ones that you are happy to live with for the rest of your life. It's not as easy as the drastic diet plan until you get into the swing of making those changes but, within a minimum of 21 days or so, they can become new habits and then they will become very easy indeed. What's more, those changes will remain with you forever and the weight will be gone for good.

Online weight loss programs
Many people feel forced to exercise just because they face people in the gym whom they would rather not see while exercising. They force themselves to imagine of some other person who has a better face and body and then perform their daily exercises. What ultimately happens is that this type of person faces failure. Always remember that whenever you feel forced to do something then if you do it the work comes to no good. If you feel uncomfortable exercising among people then go for online exercise and diet plans. For all the diet plans in the world at least one online version is sure to be available. The internet is a wealth of online tools for any dieter and is also devoid of the social stigma prevalent in a gym. The online schedule will provide you with everything starting from a diet chart to a forum section for the discussion of the success of these programs. But there are negative aspects too. You are on your own and without physical guidance. There is no-one to monitor you or tell you if you should work a bit harder or eat a bit less. This is an upper hand that a gym has over these online regimes. At the gym there is a personal trainer who will push you to push yourself harder. Also when you see others sweating, you too work harder to sweat, the atmosphere of the gym induces you to give your best. The online program will give you the schedule but not the reason for which you will feel like working out. So think before you opt for any of the two. Next is the cost of the online version as many programs charge a lot for 6-12 months, the owners of the site will not afford to work to your whim. Once you will feel it is great and the next moment you will grow lazy and lose interest, hence the online programs charge upfront. One way however you can make the most of these online plans, get print outs of the free menu plans and free routines for fitness and then use it as a guide for your daily exercise, and use all the free information you can.

Natural weight loss programs

A natural weight loss program is basically meant for everyone who is overweight. The identifier for you to undertake a weight loss program is your BMI or Body Mass Index. There are various ways in which you can find out which weight loss program is useful for you. One of those ways is finding out a good weight loss centre and you can also check online for the same. Some programs may use the technique of shifting calories for the reduction of your weight, while others will help you check your weight by balancing your meals from three large meals to four or five small meals a day. The next technique is for those who have a huge stomach. Fat reduction of the stomach is the most difficult and therefore either you should not allow yourself to procure a stomach or if you already have one then consider going for a weight loss program seriously, find out your BMI from our website www.wholebodyworkshop.com.

Pills

At present, 12-17 million people are hooked on diet pills and the figures are rising. But we are ultimately talking about a multi billion dollar industry for fat absorbing pills (just one type). That's a lot of money for something that doesn't supply you with the solution and increases damage, not just within your body, but also within your mind. There are also products that you take before meals to fill you up and reduce your appetite and these are also usually in tablet form. These may cause many problems such as wind or constipation to name only a few, not to mention giving you no solution to your problem.

Weight loss pills are the most common of the ways in which people try to reduce fat and they have been on the market for a few years now. These are however not a replacement for your diet or for that matter your exercise but it is meant to assist all the work you are doing to reduce weight. However the most important aspect of the pills is that you should never go for a random weight loss pill but should go for something that suits your body type and metabolism. Some pills will be better than others and depending on your personal circumstances you should pick your pill. There are plenty of pill types available on the market but they can all be grouped under three basic categories, and these are:

Fat burning pills

Fat burning pills are essentially designed to speed up the process of fat burning in your body. The only problem they pose is that along with speeding up the process of fat burning they also harm your health. Your ultimate aim is to lose weight but not at the cost of your health, whatever your desires you should always try to keep healthy, therefore these pills are generally not recommended for their inherent health risk.

Fat binders

These pills limit the fat absorption by your system. They prevent your body from absorbing fat from the food you eat and are somewhat safer than the fat burning pills. However these pills should be avoided by the dieter who is health conscious since like the fat burning pills they too attempt to alter the metabolic processes of your body. They also fail to address the problem of the really fat people, i.e. the problem of eating too much.

Appetite suppressor pills

The pills do exactly what its name suggests i.e. suppress your appetite for food. This product should be used if you are sure that the product is purely natural. These are perhaps the most popular of all diet pills available in the market and can be highly recommended for all. Their target is the major crisis, appetite for more and more food. It helps you control your appetite and in the process controls your diet aswell as the frequency of meals. Many appetite suppressants however are not FDA approved which would indicate that they are not safe or there is a lack of proof to say that they work.

The basic problem is that in the process of getting overweight you have actually become prone to eating more and more. You eat large quantities of food and gradually lose control over your appetite ending up overweight. If you have further added a reduced level of physical activity and exercise then you qualify for the perfect achiever of obesity. The best way to keep yourself under check is by increasing the level of your physical activity and adding an effective appetite reduction supplement to your healthy diet. The increasing popularity of the diet suppressor pill only shows that dieters now are becoming more and more conscious of their health and more knowledgeable about the diet regimes they should follow to stay slim, trim and healthy. After all health is wealth.

How do I know which advertisements to believe?

The reason why so many millions of people choose to spend their hard earned money on weight loss products and gimmicks is very simple, because of advertising. They all offer a quick fix solution to people's problems and even claim that whatever the product is, it has been scientifically proven to work. Don't you think that if it was genuine, whoever discovered it would be very close to being the world's richest person alive? I must confess, though, that the adverts and promotional stunts do actually sound appealing and I can understand why people choose that route through belief and trust. The fact is that according to the international journal of obesity, weight loss is currently a $150 billion dollar industry, and that's just in the United States and Europe alone. Can you imagine what the figure is on a global front? So do millions of people who believe that somehow, as if by waving a magic wand, they will be thin and firm?

Unwilling or unable to lose weight through diet and exercise, people turn to weight loss gimmicks ranging from pills that supposedly let them eat unlimited pasta to wearing rubber suits that make them sweat while they sleep. According to Judith Willis, editor of the United States Food and Drug Administration (FDA) Drug Bulletin, "The most current diet gimmicks of today seem to fall into two categories and they are: (1) Custom garments or body wraps that claim to "melt" fat away in a short time, and (2) Pills that supposedly curb appetites without side effects, or allow dieters to eat normally or more than normal and still lose weight. The pills are usually touted as the product of some previously undiscovered process.

Who can blame these people for being lured by the promise of losing unwanted pounds without doing anything more strenuous than popping a pill or wrapping up the offending flesh? Who can resist advertisements for body wraps that promise "to burn away fat even while you sleep," to lose 4-6 inches on the first day?

Some medical experts agree that such treatment will cause a loss of inches and perhaps pounds due to profuse perspiration. But the reductions are temporary and the fluid is soon replaced by drinking or eating. But rapid and excessive fluid loss is potentially dangerous because it can bring on severe dehydration and can upset the (homeostasis) balance of important electrolytes in the body.

Through gimmicks and lies, the consumer is being tricked into spending their hard earned money on things that, quite simply, don't work. Fortunately for you there is only one way to lose weight and successfully keep it off. You are about to discover the secret that others before you have already encountered.

YOUR HEALTH

"As you grow older, you'll find the only things you regret doing are the things you didn't do."

- Zachary Scott

How do quick weight loss attempts become unhealthy?

Things you should know first:

Risks
It will be no surprise to you that the percentage of the world in need of weight loss is extremely high, not to mention the amount of money spent on weight loss products per year is astronomically high aswell. As already mentioned, the cost is in the billions and getting higher. Once considered a problem only in high income countries, being over-weight and obese is now dramatically on the rise in low and middle income countries, particularly in urban settings. The latest World health organisation projections indicate that at least one in three of the world's adult population is overweight and almost one in ten is obese. Overweight means that they are above their natural weight and obese meaning that they are over fat.

The (W.H.O) world health organisation's latest projections indicate that, globally in 2005:

- Approximately 1.6 billion adults (age 15+) were overweight;

- At least 400 million adults were obese;

- At least 20 million children under the age of 5 years were overweight.

W.H.O further projects that by 2015, approximately 2.3 billion adults will be over-weight and more than 700 million will be obese.

Facts
Billions of people each year go on some form of diet that, quite frankly, puts the body into starvation mode, resulting in certain effects on the body, including:

- Fewer fat releasing and fat burning enzymes being released;

- Fewer hormones that tell your brain you are full are released;

- Hormones for fat burning crash;

- Muscle is cannibalised by your own body;

- Hormones controlling appetite cause ravenous cravings.

Points to note
In 1992 the British Heart Foundation was sufficiently concerned about dieting and how it increased the risk of heart disease, so much so that they produced and distributed a booklet alerting Doctors to the danger. In addition to coronary disease and heart at-tacks, there are a number of other health problems associated with yo-yo dieting. These include the previously mentioned decrease in lean tissue (including heart muscle), loss

of bone minerals, gout or gallstones, hair loss, fibrosis and tissue scarring, high blood pressure when returning to a normal diet, depression, harmful side effects of appetite depressant drugs, and shortened lifespan.

- There is no "magic bullet" when it comes to nutrition and there isn't one single diet that works for every person so you need to find an eating plan that works for you;

- Good nutrition doesn't come in a vitamin supplement and you should only take a vitamin with your doctor's recommendation because your body benefits the most when you eat healthy foods;

- Eating all different kinds of foods is best for your body. So learn to try new foods;

- Fad diets offer short term changes, but good health comes from long term effort and commitment;

- Stories from people who have used a diet program or product, especially in commercials and infomercials are advertisements; these people are usually paid to endorse what the ad is selling;

- Remember, regained weight or other problems that develop after someone has completed the diet program are never talked about in adverts;

- Filling our plates with the right food will, over time, eliminate obesity and dramatically reduce the incidence of self inflicted diseases associated with poor diet.

The diet patterns of Americans have changed rapidly over the past decade or so. The diet no longer consists of freshly made food high in nutritional value. The food no longer contains the essential carbohydrates, vitamins, minerals, water, unsaturated fat, micro nutrient, etc. on the contrary it consists of nicotine, caffeine, alcohol, preservatives, cholesterol, modified fats, starch, etc mainly because of a culture of fast food and packaged foods easy to cook that prevails among people at large. Such a diet is not only unhealthy and leads to an immediate onset of obesity because of such eating habits, but it also deprives the body of the essential nutrients that it needs. You must remember that whatever you do, you cannot possibly cheat your bodys mechanism.

The body remains unsaturated when it comes to these nutrients and tries to get them from the unhealthy food that you eat which has precious little to offer. This results in gross overeating of those foods. The behavioural patterns of Americans with respect to their money spending program are also strange. With people's incomes increasing, it has been observed that people don't use this money to buy healthy food. Rather, a huge amount has been observed to have been spent on pet food! The quality of food that they themselves eat does not go up with rise in income. On the contrary, the nutrition content in their food that is important for a proper functioning of the body reduces with the increase in income! Western weight loss institute comprises physicians, dieticians, nurses and training coaches who aim at spreading awareness among Americans regarding their food habits and exercise programs. They are a dedicated team who has looked upon obesity as a major menace plaguing the nation today and aim at reducing this problem as far as possible to eventually be able to weed it out completely. Huge national losses are also a major concern for the nation as a whole. A large number of work hours and days are lost because of some obesity related problem or another. Insurance claims are made more frequently for such problems, and companies are also spending more on their employees health, incurring large expenses.

The starvation diet is a type of dieting process in which you starve yourself to burn excess fat in your body. You are actually taking less calories so that you burn more of it off your body, but one thing that you should remember is that in this process you are restricting your diet to such a level that the low calorie intake count affects your metabolism hence forcing your body to move to a phase where you are no longer able to lose weight no matter how much you starve. To understand this process of starvation dieting we need to throw some light at what effects our slimming whims bring on our body. Usually while on a starvation diet we tend to do away with one meal in the entire day but we do not realise that this creates a crisis for the body. Firstly our body will think that we are about to take another meal so it will start to use up the blood sugar and the carbohydrates so as to lower their levels since the meal we were supposed to have would definitely increase their levels. Thus according to the body, a balance will be maintained but what the body does not know is that we are not planning on having the meal, therefore the body instead of burning up all the fat and muscle tissue, energy moves to a lower metabolism state to fight and protect the body. Ultimately what would happen if we continued to ignore our meals is that all body energy will be burnt up hence making us lethargic and slowing down our organs. Finally this would lead to something as serious as death simply because we were more concerned about our figure than about living. The solution that can be offered for losing weight rather than losing your life is moving on to a diet which will confuse your mind and body so that the metabolism stays up and at the same time you lose calories and not your muscle energy.

If you are inclined towards dieting but at the same time do not want to starve, then keep the following points in mind:

1. Why do you want to diet? Generally to lose fat;

2. What will you do to achieve your aim? Diet so that your body is comfortable with the regime but do not try to lose weight too fast as then you will go into the starvation phase;

3. What will you do to raise the metabolism of your body? Exercise to burn calories aswell as force the body to raise the metabolism, so that it is prepared to take the strain of excessive exercise.

After reading this I am sure that you will realise that your body too has certain needs which need to be fulfilled and since you are its owner you are responsible for looking after it and therefore I hope this information has helped you, even if only a tiny bit, to learn how to control and care for your body by exercise and diet. It means exactly what it reads; do not starve yourself to lose weight. I am sure that like most other people you too believe that starvation is the only way to lose weight. However it is very important for you to not skip your meals as the saying goes: "Eat breakfast like a king, eat a nutritious lunch, and eat your evening meal like a pauper."

Starving has one major side effect that it makes the body switch to the "survival mode". The metabolism slows down and all the body fat will be burnt so that we stay alive at the cost of losing all the energy of the body. You might wonder how the body has learnt to switch to this emergency mode so for your knowledge, the mechanisms have been learnt by the human body as a means of adaptation since in ancient times certain periods of the year were fruitless and therefore the body got rarely anything or entirely nothing to survive on. But this hardly means that we can also do the same now because at that time it was adaptation which has stayed with us to save our lives for a certain period but it will not save you if you starve for months with the hope of slimming down. To better illustrate the point let me say - "have you ever seen a skinny bear go into hibernation?" I am sure you would say no therefore please eat regularly and properly.

Why are most weight loss advertisements unhealthy myths?

Obesity is turning out to be a major menace all over the world. With more and more people leading busy lifestyles, the kind of attention they can give to themselves and their bodies is slowly decreasing and as a result obesity takes over. Fast weight loss measures are rapidly being sought simply because of the busy lifestyles that people, at large, lead. It is generally when someone is faced with some major event such as a holiday or wedding that they realise that they must lose all those unnecessary pounds. The lives of people these days comprise working, eating insensibly and watching the television whenever there is free time at hand. After a busy day's work, working out is something that people do not want to do, as they wish to 'relax'. The thought of beginning a diet and exercise regime from the next weekend always crosses ones mind, just that the 'next weekend' never really arrives. This has led to various people and companies claiming that they have just what the public at large needs, that is, some magic potion that will help you reduce those precious pounds before you realise it, and the best way to go about campaigning is of course through the television. Magazines are also filled with advertisements regarding fast weight reduction methods by simply popping a couple of pills a day. The shiny happy faces, and slim body structures accompanying the products are enough to put anyone in the loop.

As much as we wish this was true, that by just applying some magic cream one could lose weight without any effort, it is not. This is only one tiny scheme in a pool of various schemes floating to get money out of gullible consumers always looking for easy and quick fix remedies to their problems. The worst part is that there may be people who have actually lost weight by falling for such products. You may know some of them personally and may believe their word for it when they say the product has actually worked. But you must also know that what they have lost is not fat from their

16

body, but merely water. This is, needless to say, unhealthy. As we know, the human body is a divine machine. That is to say, it has its own mechanisms and everything within the body is networked and interconnected so as to form this one big chain which allows everyday functioning of the body. The body has its own habits and its own clock. Suddenly you decide to go on a diet or pop some unhealthy pills, the body does not obviously know that this was coming and takes this as a rude shock to its very being. These pills are meant to reduce water in the body but the body, having a strong survival streak will not let that happen, so what it does to conserve the energy that those pills are bent at sucking out, is to slow down its metabolism. Once the metabolism is slowed down, it means that any food you eat will not get as easily and as fully processed as it used to be before. The food will not break down into simpler substances like carbohydrates, energy, etc as easily, and will get stored under the layers of your skin as fat. Therefore, once after your fast weight loss routine if you start having food again, the efficiency of the body to process food will have reduced and therefore rapid weight gain will be observed. Also, rapid weight loss means that the muscles under your skin have just shrunk without giving the skin a chance to adjust hence why there is loose skin and stretch marks.

Under normal and healthy circumstances, the average amount of weight loss someone can achieve in a week is about 2-3 pounds. Fast ways of losing weight by expecting to lose 10-15 pounds a week is not only difficult, but it is ridiculous to even think of, given that you plan to go about this in a normal manner by eating healthy and exercising. It is also extremely difficult to gain 10-15 in one week, but if you have gained that much weight, then you have been consistently overeating without exercising regularly. Therefore, there's no point trying to wish those pounds away in a jiffy. Believing in all those advertisements that flood your television and your mailbox is idiotic. The creators of these products and advertisements have done their market research well and they know that people like you and me are on a consistent lookout for fast and easy weight reduction measures and that is exactly what they tell back to you. This is a sensitive topic to billions of people who in desperation, will do all that is necessary.

You are bent on losing your weight and also as fast as possible and for that you have fixed your diet chart, hope to follow it diligently and lose those love handles as fast as you can. But you may also be wondering about the amount of weight that you can lose in just a week's time. In this case something you should always remember is that if you lose weight too fast then it can be dangerous for you. There are many things that can affect your weight loss program. For example your family history and genetics can play a major role in determining whether you can lose weight effectively. Side by side the amount of weight lost by you is also determined by the amount of exercise you do to lose weight. Major effects can be put on your weight loss schedule also by your metabolism capacity and the rate at which your body burns calories. Theoretically, human bodies are capable of losing upto 20 pounds at the most in one week however much of that weight will be water lost by the body in that one week. This means that you run the risk of putting on weight as soon as you do away with your diet schedule.

The mechanism which makes the weight loss theory possible is the adaptation undergone by the body during ancient times when there used to be lack of food for a specific period. Nature has endorsed us with this way of protecting our body against too much weight loss and therefore whenever the calorie count of the body decreases drastically then the body compensates for it by the reduction of the rate of metabolism. This is actually an explanation for the fact that certain human beings can lose weight only up to a certain extent and no more in spite of trying very hard. If you are planning on losing weight fast then one thing that I think I should bring to your notice is that in this process of frenzied weight loss you will actually be jeopardising your health by initiating the appearance of gall stones, loosening your skin and a tremendous free fall of your weight. But the worst thing of all that will happen to you is that you will gain weight as rapidly as you had lost it so what is the use? Furthermore after you have achieved whatever weight you wanted to, you will fall into bad eating habits and hence ruin your system, therefore think again before you make a decision.

The point that had been made at the end of the last section that of a bad eating habit after a period of deprivation of food needs to be elaborated a bit. Firstly you will be very much tempted to further starve yourself since you will not feel the urge or need to eat due to a long period of doing the same, keeping yourself from eating and as a result suffer from anorexia. Secondly if you feel the urge to eat then you will be eating so much that you will turn yourself into a patient suffering from bulimia. Therefore lose weight only under medical supervision and not on a whim, preventing yourself from harming your body. There are a number of ways that you can undertake to lose your weight but still stay healthy and not harm your body, therefore follow healthy and safe procedures. Add exercise to your regime, walk, jog, and workout anything to speed up your weight loss process but abstain from methods which break your body system down. Do you know that you can lose as much as 2 pounds by just walking for one week? So stop torturing your body and start following a reasonable healthy diet coupled with lots of exercise and water intake which will keep you fit and at the same time help you lose weight too.

When is the right time to see your doctor?

Do you feel that you have an eating disorder? Do you not feel full even after eating a sufficient quantity of food, do you seem to eat a lot but despite that, you lose weight, do you take laxatives or resort to vomiting to compensate for the extra calories that you have taken in, are you always chronically depressed? If the answer to any of these questions is yes, then it is advisable that you must see a doctor at once. Most of the time we forget that sometimes we eat not because of necessity but out of sheer habit, it does happen that no matter how full we are we still carry a bag of popcorn with us to the movie hall, the same is the case when we are watching television at home, we do not open that bag of potato chips because we are hungry, we do so only because we are habituated to do so. People who eat in excess or have the dietary disorder bulimia, do not have any sense of control, they cannot help but eat a large quantity of food at a single sitting. People who are most prone to this disorder are the people who have tried their hand at dieting but have failed miserably; such people have very low self esteem. There are many similarities between bulimia and anorexia, the most common being the cause. There seems to be a common occurrence of sexual and/or physical and emotional abuse in direct relation to both eating disorders (though not all people living with

18

eating disorders are survivors of abuse). There also seems to be a direct connection in some people to clinical depression. The eating disorder sometimes causes the depression or the depression can lead to the eating disorder.

All in all, eating disorders are very complex emotional issues. Though they may seem to be nothing more than a dangerously obsessive weight concern on the surface, for most men and women suffering with an eating disorder there are deeper emotional conflicts to be resolved. Another class of people who are prone to eating disorder are the people who are addicted to a certain thing and are trying to quit. For example in case of chronic smokers who are trying to quit, there is a chance that they indulge in food, this is mainly because they need to keep their hands and mouth occupied, Most of the time these people overcome the want of nicotine, with the pleasure of food. According to many doctors, people who are prone to depression resort to food and this gives them emotional support which in turn helps them to forget about their depression for a while. It has been proved that in many cases it is not just the psychological factor that causes us to over-eat, it is the brain that prompts us to indulge in overeating. People who have low levels of serotonin (a chemical in the brain) often crave carbohydrates no matter how much they eat, the same is the case with people who have a tumour or people who have injured their hypothalamus section of the brain.

There are certain glandular problems also, that causes us to over-eat, an overactive thyroid gland can cause us to increase the metabolic rate leaving the body to crave for food, and also in case of untreated diabetes the body tries to generate fuel for the body in the form of food. There are certain medicines mainly pain relievers and also anti depressants that increases the appetite for food, the one medicine that is notorious for increasing the appetite is Cortisone.

The main reason why people are overweight these days is due to overeating, this means taking in more calories than what is needed by the body, on an average our body needs 1500 to 2000 calories but in the course of our day we end up taking a lot more of these calories, thus this leads to weight gain.

Here we have eight causes that lead to weight gain:

1. Skipping meals: when you eat a proper meal your body will not crave food till it is the time to eat at the next meal, but when you skip a meal your body will overcompensate for it and you will end up eating more than what you would have eaten at the next meal, thus it is a disaster to skip a meal as you tend to reverse the affect of dieting;

2. Lack of rest and sleep: when you are sleep starved you lose control over yourself, you end up eating a lot more than you would normally have and you generally eat more sugar which leads to weight gain. This is a common phenomenon which happens at the end of the week, you eat a lot more sugar than on a Monday in which you are well rested due to the weekend;

3. Big portions: most of the time we do not eat as to how much should suffice our hunger but we eat as much as there is on our plate. In case there is a lot of food on our plate we end up eating that without thinking whether we actually need to eat it or not. We should take smaller portions on our plate, preferably go for smaller plates. We know that we do not need more than 2000 calories and as such we should divide it into six, that is three meals and three snacks and thus divide our calories in manageable slots;

4. Keep a check on carbohydrates: most of the time we eat very heavy food, french fries and bagels to name but a few, these foods are excessively rich in carbohydrates and thus these should be best avoided, try and make a note of certain items that are a part of your daily diet and hence causes your weight gain;

5. Food commercials: there are certain food commercials that are a great turn on and same is the case with food smells, as these food smells make us forget everything and just makes us go for the forbidden food. This happens mainly when you are passing by a hamburger stall or any fast food chain;

6. Lack of fibre: our body needs fibre to fill it up, it is important that we take in enough fibre. In case we do not our body compensates for it by taking in more of carbohydrates;

7. Artificial sweeteners: there are artificial sweeteners like saccharin and we over indulge in food having saccharin because we feel that because it is artificial but we forget that overall the food itself is high in calories;

8. Stress: stress causes us to over-eat, in case of stressful situations it is advisable that you snack on low calorie foods such as carrots, cucumber etc, also try and exercise regularly as this will reduce stress, also it is important to keep the right attitude and try and avoid stress as much as possible.

You may not be accustomed to discussing your feelings or personal problems with your doctor. Keep in mind that the doctor cannot know you're strained, disturbed or anxious just by seeing you. Be honest with him or her, and note such emotions. The doctor will ensure that other health problems are not the cause of your physical symptoms. If other health problems are not the basis of the symptoms, then both you and your doctor can deal with the emotional reasons of these signs. The doctor's suggestions will treat the bodily warning signs. Meanwhile, both you and he can tackle your emotional condition. If your intense negative feelings prevent you from enjoying life and do not disappear, then it is imperative for a medical consultation. These are the signs of "major depression". A medical disease treated with individualised counselling, holistic therapies or medicines (or all) is referred to as depression.

Binge eating

A form of eating disorder where the patient impulsively overeats or eats more than the normal requirements is called binge eating. Their actions and appearance point to getting insufficient food, as if they are never full. The normal symptoms of binge eating are: eating rapidly suggesting in need of command, recurring incidents of excessive eating, eating secretly, and hoarding and hiding food. During and after eating the binge eater feels miserable, guilty and sickened. To alleviate tension, the person binge eats and they sense the necessity for a strong willpower. Apart from feeling useless and disheartened, they are also a perfectionist. They try hard to avoid fights and to gratify people as they feel repelled at body size. Possibly, they would attempt to solve their dilemma of binge eating, alone. Usually, this fails to work making the disorder worse. This persists till a support group of family or friends realise the situation and ask for help. Trouble doing physical exercise or walking, having unusual levels of exhaustion, blood sugar, having heart and blood pressure difficulty and joint problems are the physical signs of a binge eater. Spells of eating huge amounts of food in a short time span without considering hunger or fullness are typical characteristics of a binge eater. They would admit to being unchecked while eating enormously. The quantity of food eaten will result in guilt, disgust and shame.

Cures for compulsive eating and food cravings

You can eliminate food cravings by control and eating small amounts of food instead of forbidding yourself of food. How do you cope with your repeated cravings of eating treats that will ruin your weight loss attempts? Eating dense low-energy foods like vegetables, fruits and soups as shown by many studies, maintain satiety and reduces energy intake. A more successful weight loss strategy advising individuals in a clinical trial is eating portions of low-energy, dense foods than fat reduction coupled with restriction of portion sizes. Satiety can be enhanced and hunger controlled even restricting energy intake for weight on consuming fulfilling portions of low-energy dense foods (Ello-Martin, JA, 2005).

You can do the following things before you "give in" to unplanned cravings:

1. Have a glass of water or a cup of herbal or fruit tea when you feel like eating. Drink something before eating as maybe you were only thirsty, and not hungry;

2. Even if it's another floor in your office building, walk briskly. Remind your body's goals while doing a few stretches;

3. If you don't want to lose that fresh and clean feeling, carry your toothbrush and paste with you everywhere to brush your teeth;

4. Ask yourself if you are actually hungry, if you still really want the food;

5. Decide on your real temptation after examining the situation. Why did you have a sudden urge to eat something? Were offered food visible to you? Did a

walk make you pass the fridge? Did boredom strike you with your current activity? You will realise that wanting the food was nothing more than an impulse;

6. Think about what will truly satisfy your hunger after judging if you are physically hungry. What do you need to eat something crunchy, a bit of sweet, a little something to nibble, or a something salty or something filling? To satisfy any type of hunger, you will find a healthy alternative. For unhealthy treats, keep healthy substitutes at hand.

If everything unfortunately fails, eat the food. But, enjoy the food you really desperately wanted without a guilty conscience and eat it slowly. Exercise a little extra and have smaller portions throughout the day to compensate for your craving to get things back on track.

How can you improve your emotional health and wellbeing?

Firstly, try to identify your emotions and the causes behind their occurrence. You can manage your emotional health by identifying the grounds for stress, sadness and worry in your life.

Emotionally healthy people are conscious of their behaviours, feelings and thoughts. The stress and problems of their lives are negligible due to their knowledge of coping with them. They have fulfilling relationships and are positive about themselves. The things that can interrupt your emotional state and make you strongly feel sad, anxious or stressed include:

- Being fired from your job;

- A child leaving or returning home;

- Coping with a loved one's demise;

- Marrying or divorcing;

- Enduring a disease or an injury;

- Being professionally promoted;

- Undergoing financial troubles;

- Shifting to a new house or giving birth.

Both "good" and "bad" changes can be equally stressful.

The frequently termed "mind/body connection" is your body's response to your manner of thinking, feeling and acting. Your body attempts to inform you that things are unsuitable when you are worried or apprehensive. For instance, a particularly stressful event like a loved one's death can lead to the growth of a stomach ulcer or high blood pressure.

The following physical signs indicate an imbalanced emotional health:

- Back ache;

- Altered appetite;

- Upper body pain;

- Diarrhoea or constipation;

- Dried up mouth;

- Intense weariness;

- Common aches;

- Headaches;

- High blood pressure;

- Insomnia – sleeplessness;

- Dizziness;

- Palpitations - feeling hurried heartbeats;

- Sexual troubles;

- Shortness of breath;

- Rigid neck;

- Sweating;

- Troubling stomach;

- Change in weight.

Your body's immunity can deteriorate due to a poor emotional situation, making you susceptible to colds and other infections in emotionally turbulent times. At these times you will probably not take appropriate care of your health. You might not wish to exer-

cise, devour nutritious food or take the doctors prescribed medicines. Another indication of poor emotional health is the abuse of tobacco, alcohol or other drugs.
Express your feelings in suitable ways, because bottling up negative feelings can be worse if they are creating physical ailments. It is perfectly fine to inform your nearest and dearest about your source for concern. Nevertheless, understand that your loved ones may be powerless to aid in the proper dealing of your feelings. When these occur, take the advice and support of an outsider from the circumstances i.e. like a counsellor, your family doctor, holistic therapist or a religious guide to aid improvement in your emotional health.

Live a balanced life and don't attempt to think about situations that raise negative feelings like troubles at home, work or school. You do not have to act happy when you are emotionally unstable. Try to emphasise on the good things in your life, aswell as deal with depressing feelings. You might want to keep a journal to record the things that make you smile and feel at peace. Your quality of life can be improved and your fitness can recover, as proved by studies. You have to search for ways to get rid of stressful and overpowering negative things in your life, so take out time for things you get pleasure from. Calm your mind and body, as your emotions can be balanced through constructive methods of relaxation like meditation. It is a type of guiding thoughts, available in several manifestations. For instance, you may meditate through exercise, breathing deeply and stretching. You can take your holistic therapists, doctor's guidance on means of relaxation. Take care of your body to ensure excellent emotional health, this can be by a regular schedule of eating nutritious food, sleeping as much as necessary and exercising to mitigate hidden tension. Avoid overeating and drug or alcohol abuse, using these creates other multiple troubles, like those of health and family.

How do you maintain a healthy weight?

Benefits
The benefits of you losing weight personally will be very similar to the next person's benefits. For example, you'll both be looking good, feeling good, be able to do more things physically and have an improved quality of life, including raised self esteem and less depression. But just look at all the health benefits there are from you losing weight. You reduce your risk of heart disease; your cholesterol comes down, particularly the bad type (LDL), while the heart protective good cholesterol (HDL) goes up significantly. Weight loss can reduce the risk of osteoarthritis, gout and even some cancers including endometrial, breast and colon, to name but a few. All of these conditions can cause premature death and substantial disability. In addition to all of these benefits, blood pressure and sugar levels come down, which is particularly helpful for diabetics. Plus, there are all the side benefits, such as less tiredness, back pain, joint pain, sweating, breathlessness, snoring, infertility, menstrual irregularities, urinary leakage, etc. The only sure, safe way to lose your excess weight and keep it off is Mother Nature's way. Your body has built-in, natural fat burners but, through bad nutrition, these fat-burners become dysfunctional, dormant or plain lazy. That's why you're overweight and the only way you can lose weight and keep it off is to get your natural fat burners functioning normally and at peak efficiency again. This book will show you how.

Consider this small example: If you don't take proper care of your car on a regular basis, if you refuse to fuel it whenever the need be, or if you turn a blind eye to signals, would your car look good or run properly? No! The same applies for your body, which you must maintain properly at all times.

Start with changing your mindset about dieting. People often confuse dieting as being a tool to lose weight, which is completely false. What is needed is a healthy level of weight, to attain which you have to work and maintain yourself regularly. As you always have to look after your car to ensure a smooth run, you must take care of your body at all times aswell.

Body mass index (BMI) & health risk
The BMI predicts body fat and disease risk better than the popular height/weight tables. A high BMI links to increased risk of death from all causes.

Certain people should not use BMI to infer being overweight or relative disease risk. These people are competitive athletes, body builders, pregnant or lactating women, growing children or sedentary elderly adults. Body mass index (BMI) represents the ratio of body mass (weight) to stature (height) squared.

BMI = Body mass divided by stature – squared (a calculator will be placed on the website for you)

In June of 1998 the first federal guidelines were released for identifying, evaluating and treating overweight and obesity.

The classifications on BMI are as follows:

Classification	BMI Score	Health risk
Underweight	18.5	
Normal	18.5-24.9	
Overweight	25.0-29.9	Minimal 25.0 / Low 25-27 / Moderate 27-30
Obesity class I	30.0-34.9	High 30-<35
Obesity class II	35.0-39.9	Very high 35-<40
Extreme obesity	>40.0	>40 Extremely high

YOUR MIND

"Change your thoughts and you change your world."

- Norman Vincent Peale

How can your mind and body work together for permanent success?

In earlier times, a few physicians dismissed digestive problems without any symptom of organic illness as being psychological. Scientists now think the mind and the body's operations are interconnected, as opposed to the past. Complex links are noted by doctors between the digestive and nervous systems. Anything that influences one will concern the other due to the continuous exchange of electrical and chemical messages between the two. The original evidence relating the therapeutic power of the mind to our bodies is conveyed to us every day. Prayer or any kind of mediation genuinely soothes us, which in turn may assist us to face our routine stressors. Nowadays fitness specialists add onto this notion, essentially informing you which parts of your body and muscles are accountable, or "connected" to which aspects of your daily living. This translates into physiology and psychology being attached together. For those planning your own workouts, this is a good subject to investigate more closely.

The western world is currently faced with a critical situation of succumbing to the epidemic of obesity and blood sugar. The boat is sinking as it is weighed down with psychological barriers related to weight loss by loading it with statistics of grams, calories and pounds. You want to feel better and stronger by losing some weight, but you do not know the right path to being successful. In order to prevent your general health from going down the drains, you must adopt these two steps:

Step-1) Get rid of your hang ups!
It is not really difficult for you to start exercising. You should concentrate more upon the positive aspect instead of unconsciously resisting them getting better. Exercise resistance, refers to the conscious or unconscious blocking out of participation in a program which demands regular activities. As studies show, this might result from bitter past experiences which turn individuals into being apathetical towards exercise and healthy food. These prevent people from following an exercise program religiously more often than not. The root of resenting exercise travels deeper than just disliking the effort it takes to carry them out. Resentment only makes a rebel out of us, and people generally tend to think that the exercises, instead of being rigorous and demanding so much hard work, are actually supposed to make them feel at their best. What you really need to do is accept exercise as a part of your life, as something that is as important as brushing your teeth or brushing your hair. Resentment comes hand in hand with denial, vanity and laziness.

Initial failures must be interpreted positively, as we fail only when we don't start. Success can never be measured by virtue of its numerical or statistical value, but by the ways in which you keep growing in due course of the process. You must never be afraid of failure. If you take a little more time than others to finally make it through, it is not considered to be a failed effort, not even under comparative circumstances. You must also keep in mind that perfection can never really be achieved permanently and is but an illusion. You must never compare yourself with the performances of others either. Goals, no matter how many you achieve or score, will always be there, and what really counts is improving yourself since you are the best judge of your own standards.

The psychology of weight loss has both negative aswell as positive sides, however, when it comes to the negative aspect you might overburden yourself with high expectations, which ultimately leads to setting yourself up for failure. This can ultimately prove to be extremely harmful.

Step-2) Changing the foolish beliefs about life, food and exercise
You need to unearth the roots of the things you are concerned with, and you need to come to terms with your attitude towards exercise and eating. A lot of people live under the illusion that they are very much acquainted with their thought procedures, while reality eludes them.

If you really want to change your food and exercise habits, you need to get to the heart of the matter and discover the reasons behind your behaviour. In this context your belief and faith has a huge and important role to play. Your belief and faith stems from your core values which influences an essential part of your life. You can overcome a great deal of your limitations if you can adjust your beliefs when required, which lie deep within you. Your beliefs can stand against your successful carrying out of exercise programs, and they need to be changed if necessary. You can never have everything easy, and to get to where the situation needs you to be, it takes a great deal of time, energy and effort on your part. You must look inside in order to overcome the psychological barriers which stand in your way of losing weight. It is high time that you either do what you must, or be prepared to face the consequences. It is not that you need to be scared, you just need to be systematic in your approach and calculate properly what you are required to do in reality, and do not just rely on your faith or luck. Get out there and do what you have to. Make exercising a part of your daily life, and be positive in your psychological responses to weight loss. Getting in shape is more of an internal process than it is an external one. When we get the internal stuff right... the external change is merely a positive by-product.

How does food affect your mind?

The human mind is fragile. The entire system is interconnected through this mass of neurons and this connection is so sensitive that even if one link of the entire chain is missing, the connection snaps, the mind goes wobbly. The mind is considered the strength of the human body, but at the same time it is extremely vulnerable to all sorts of attacks. A simple fever can make the mind go blank and during very high fever several people say all sorts of things they have no recollection of when they are back to normal. This is because they have lost a hold on their minds. The mind, more so than the body needs proper nutrition for its proper functioning. Food must be eaten not only for a healthy body, but also for a healthy and well functioning mind. Caffeine, nicotine, chocolate overdose, etc cause the mind even greater damage than they cause the body. Such food substances cause havoc in the entire neurological system. The neurotransmitters may get blocked because such foods are certainly not what they need and therefore are not welcomed by them.
"Holistic" thinkers have existed for a long time, constantly repeating the philosophy that the body and the mind are inextricably interconnected, and that any tiny trouble in one necessarily affects the other. However this philosophy was considered just the mus-

28

ing of some men who thought themselves wise. In the 70s and the 80s however, science discovered a connection path called neurotransmitters and realised that the philosophy of those ancient thinkers was necessarily true. Even scientists now believe and propagate the thought that the mind and the body are linked in such inextricable terms that it is difficult to separate one's activities from another's. Here's where you can get a brief look into the neurotransmitter model that scientists came up with. First, to understand what these neurotransmitters actually do, they are responsible for maintenance of the alertness chemicals and the calming chemical. These two chemicals are absolutely indispensable in the human body and the human mind. They are responsible for the thought process to happen smoothly. Now, the two main macro nutrients in the body are proteins and carbohydrates, and these nutrients transmit the neurotransmitters making it possible to generate the alertness and the calming chemicals in an effective manner, enabling the mind to be energetic and calm in face of stress. The nutrition intakes are all complementary to one another. The amino acids in protein foods are of various kinds, and these vie for access to the brain which helps create a balanced system within the body. But if a large amount of carbohydrate food is taken in with proteins, then the starch in the carbohydrates takes up the amino acids for itself, preventing the amino acids from reaching the brain. Eating food only rich in proteins causes an overdose of amino acids resulting in lethargy, therefore and ideal combination would be protein food accompanied with a little carbohydrate food aswell. This keeps the mind alert and focused.

The following is a brief but comprehensive combination of nutrients if taken in, helping the functioning of the mind in a better and healthier way:

- The mind needs to be calm and alert along with energetic in order to function well. This is a balanced state of mind where both calmness aswell as energy of the mind is equally important. Therefore sufficient quantities of proteins and carbohydrates are what you need. Therefore combinations of grain and beans, or fish and rice, or bread and hummus, or a chicken sandwich can produce the nutrients necessary for such a state of mind;

- For a mind that needs to be strongly energetic, less carbohydrates must be consumed and more of protein. Proteins mainly are energy generating and carbohydrates are responsible for taking away some of the amino acids that generate energy. Therefore consuming less of carbohydrate will prevent this from happening. For this combination, eating beans and veggies, or scallops and broccoli, or fish and salad, etc prove useful;

- For an intensely calm mind, more of carbohydrates and little of protein are ideal. Carbohydrates cause calmness. If more of protein is consumed then the energies of the carbohydrate will be directed towards the amino acids that the proteins produce and the carbohydrate will not affect the mind's calmness that well. In such a case you can eat foods such as: bananas, whole grains and veggies, pasta in garlic and oil, breakfast cereal and crackers.

Eating due to emotional needs

First of all it is important that you accept the fact that food has the power to help you cope through very difficult situations of stress, thus it is important that you understand that your body craves for food, not only when you need food but also when you need any emotional comfort. Thus, it is important that you learn to segregate the call of your body for food from the call of your body for food to get emotional satisfaction. Secondly, it is important to understand the type of pattern that you associate with food, for example, you should maintain a food diary and write down all what you have eaten for a week. Make sure that you keep a note of everything you ate and what you felt after eating them. Also write down what made you eat the food that you would not have otherwise eaten. After a week try and find a pattern in the food habits. You may find out that you eat the most when you are depressed or lonely. Maybe you eat most when you anticipate trouble at the work place, this way you can actually find out what your problem is and where it lies. You can try and find an alternative solution to your problem rather than binging on food. In case your career is what is causing you stress, you can take the help of a career counselor, or you can go out and join a club especially if you are feeling lonely. Another factor that causes you to overeat is stress, and more than half of the people who are overweight admit that they overeat when they are stressed. They admit that in situations of stress, they eat unhealthy food, such as they go in for a pizza whereas they could have easily consumed a fruit smoothie.

Understand your physical and emotional reasons for food

Most people on a diet or a mission to lose weight get to a point where they hate food and wonder why it is controlling the way they look and feel. This attitude of course becomes one of resentment and an inner sadness, which clearly affects the emotional state of each individual.

Physical reasons for food:

- Not eating enough volume of food which leaves you with an empty tummy too soon after a meal;

- Not eating enough calories, leaving you with low blood sugar and a need to eat pretty quickly to correct it;

- Eating foods that are high in fast releasing carbohydrate or sugar (high GI foods), which give a spike to your blood sugar and a rapid decline as your body tries to correct it.

Emotional reasons for food:

- Delicious foods are all around you, making it difficult to resist;

- Feeling down and eating for comfort;

- Eating to plug a gap inside because you literally feel empty;

- Eating because you are bored, which is the case with many people who are hungry all the time, as eating literally passes the time.

Life is sweeter without refined sweets but when you are stressed you will eat sweeter, fatty foods and you will ultimately increase your appetite for carbohydrates and fat.

What effect does mood swings and stress have on your eating habits?

Eating is a very common stress buster, and at a time when you feel stressed out, you not only eat more, but eat in a very fast manner, thus sending signals to your body that you don't have enough time, though reality may be otherwise. In fact, even our bodies demand certain kind of foods like sugar and fat, during those times, since they can be consumed pretty fast, so under stress, a healthy diet takes a complete backseat.
It is important to note that you must not let your body be under stress for a long period of time since it is not good for health. Food gives you relief for a temporary time but it does not solve the problem. Though there is a direct link between eating and stress, you must draw a line by making a new eating pattern. For instance, after a day of hard work if you feel stressed out and move on straight into the kitchen to eat something, try changing this routine by heading for a quick shower immediately after returning home. If you feel like eating something even after the shower, do so. But by following such a routine for many days, you will surely find that you are making good progress in controlling your eating habits and keeping them under check.

Recognise what sparks off your binging exercise
Circumstances aswell as feelings that lead all the people to gorge more than required are:

Communal
This involves consuming food in the presence of others. Like, other people might persuade you to gorge or you might go on eating so as to fall in with others or you might argue with someone or even feel certain meagerness in front of others.

Psychological
A person often binges because he or she is stressed, worried, alone, hurt or annoyed, therefore eating becomes a manner to "fill the void."

Circumstantial
This involves consuming food whenever the chance presents itself, like at a restaurant, a café, when going past a bakery or even when randomly checking out a billboard flashing a picture of some food.

Contemplation or opinion
This is when a person binges either because he or she suffers from some kind of an inferiority complex or when they simply think of reasons to binge.

Bodily aspects
This includes eating due to some disorder in the physical body system such as consuming a lot of food as a person has not eaten for a long time or maybe binging to keep away some physical ache.

Maintain a diary that will show every time that you have had food and also the reasons why you have eaten at that specific hour. It will keep the emotional state, aswell as the physiological state that you were in when you had your meal. This will help you to comprehend what exactly sets off your binging process. Also you will, very swiftly, observe a kind of routine to your eating habits

Breaking the habit
Firstly you need to recognise the thing that prompts the binging desire. Well this surely is not adequate to transform your food habits because your food habits have already become a conventional way with you. What you need to do now is prevent this from happening, and secondly, you need to indulge in other activities. The best way to get away from the binging experiences is to get into other habits and this works out most proficiently when it is carried out after quite a number of such lows. Divert your attention to something else when you feel the drive to eat, you can try any of the following: check out the programs on television, peruse a book or journal, switch on the music system, take a walk, breathe in fresh air, converse with a friend, play some games, give yourself the pleasure of a warm bath, go for a run, indulge in some household activity, check the clothes for washing, take the dog out for a walk or maybe swim, comb your hair, clean your teeth or basically do anything that you wish except rushing to the kitchen to eat. Continue the work till you get over the desire to gorge.

Tackling the issue
It is not a good idea to substitute your binging disorder with some other custom as you cannot tackle your depression in this manner. You can deal with your emotional problem by indulging in:

- Handling strain;

- Calming down methods;

- Contemplation;

- Workouts;

- Counselling in groups;

- Counselling alone.

These methods not only deal with the depression but also enable you to find a remedy to the root cause and also you can learn to deal in a better and more effective manner.

Pat yourself on the back

Once you are successful in following a healthy diet and gradually getting accustomed to the various methods of keeping up and adding more methods to grow thin, stop to appreciate your efforts. Feel good about having met your diet aims because we always end up doing those things that are imposed. Shop for the clothes that have caught your attention, go on a trip or even allow yourself a great massage because you have done well. These things will inspire you to adhere to your healthy diet even more, but it is not only about breaking old habits and building new ones that require quite a lot of commitment, as it is those commitments that have to be reconstructed and modified, not just each and every day, but every hour.

It is for the initial pain and torture that most of the New Year's Resolutions do not last beyond January, whatever the resolution may be, be it regarding losing weight, quitting smoking, watching less TV, or going back to school. All of them are quite formidable and huge changes in life, and they require not only dedication, but also self discipline. Making new habits and breaking old habits include anything and everything, from trying to refrain from a serious addiction of heroin to even, say, trying to cut down on negative thinking. One thing should be kept in mind: whenever there are some new habits in progress they will get simpler and easier with time. That is, in other words, once the initial torture of trying to incorporate new habits and breaking the old ones is over, you will, certainly, love your new way of life.

How can you achieve a positive mindset in order to lose weight?

Keep in mind what you would like to hear about yourself from other people, i.e. do you really need someone to fill you with positive thoughts and inspirations? Wouldn't you be able to do it yourself? Build your own positive thoughts, and tell yourself everything that you would like to hear from others and repeat those thoughts to yourself everyday. You might find it strange initially, but after a while, you might not even feel that you're doing so. In such a case, the maintenance of a healthy weight will be a near reality, and not a distant dream.

Resisting temptation

Researchers from Duke University, the University of Southern California, and the University of Pennsylvania found out what can resist temptation in college students is that asking them about their vices, and thus making them completely conscious and aware of that. The researchers said: "We demonstrate that asking consumers to report their expectations regarding how often they will perform a vice behaviour increases the incidence of these behaviours." It is difficult to resist temptation if one thinks about that which he is trying to resist.The study participants thought of succumbing, so inevitably they did and the main reason why resisting temptation was so difficult for them was actually their own thought processes.

Research shows us that the more somebody talks about a product, the more chances the consumer buys that product. Even harmless questions about that product will lessen the resistance to temptation. In other words, the products which people would not normally buy they would end up buying if the product is talked about. This is how the law of

Attraction works and the thoughts of the consumers are translated into action. It goes without saying that these were even more evident in people who had lesser self control. What's the payoff in succumbing to temptation? Is there a benefit in resisting temptation? There is certainly some kind of payoff which one would get as a price of resisting temptation; otherwise nobody would go for that. At the same time it is true that to resist eating a whole bag of Oreos is not half as satisfying as eating the cookies. Eating them would allow him to avoid the otherwise apparent feelings like sadness, disappointment, or loss.

In a similar fashion, to resist drinking in the night is not satisfactory, while drinking will help to forget childhood traumatic experiences, along with it helps to deal with pain, or even to suppress feelings of shame or guilt. Likewise cutting oneself is much more satisfying than to resist cutting, for that allows shift of focus to the physical pain, and thus diverts that from the inner emotional turmoil. Behind each and every action we take, there is some reason, even if that reason is not very apparent. So what is advisable is that when one is struggling with temptation, he should try to look beyond the apparent, and see what the ultimate result is behind succumbing to temptation or resisting temptation. It should be kept in mind that resisting temptation will eventually lead to a happy and healthy life. The best way to resist temptation is to turn temptation around, that is, it is better to start eating fresh fruits and vegetables, or going out to walk or jog, instead of thinking about eating chocolate chip cookies. Likewise, instead of thinking about gorging, it is better to focus on the other ways in which the money can be spent. These alternate ways eventually help in resisting temptation, as instead of surfing the net, and screwing the sleep cycle, it is always better to think about the benefits of good sleep, or spending quality time with family and friends and with time, as one would learn more about resisting temptation, the easier it would be. Rewarding yourself is one wonderful option of resisting temptation, you may bribe yourself with a movie, a trip to the beach, watching a play or a performance once you are able to resist temptation. There should be an internal focus of control that you need to empower yourself.

How can you overcome the "triggers" for overeating?

Boredom - When you are bored or have nothing interesting to look forward to, you eat. A preferred pastime on being bored and lonely at home is watching TV or constantly on the computer. It is hard to resist the refrigerator when the food advertisements run 200 images hourly into our cerebral cortex. View nature shows or TV without advertisements, if food commercials are a trigger.

Beat it by: leave some healthy food such as cut vegetables in the fridge, if you are habituated to eat anything out of the refrigerator.

Feeling deprived - You desire the foods that you love even further when you feel denied of them. Evasion of entire food groups and limiting dieting are an outcome of the media's stress on thinness as ideal. The restrictions break your plan to eat a prohibited food due to the powerful stimuli of the visibility and accessibility of the shunned food. After this, you feel devastating guilt and low self esteem, and to overcome this, you are forced to eat the avoided food.

Beat it by: Through healthy eating and training your lifestyle, aim to balance both calorie input and output out of a genuine care for your own health. Note: There is no danger to eat high fat foods in moderation.

Feeling disgust or hatred with your body - In spite of the assault of preposterous body ideals, women are unable to accept their bodies, and this is one of the many reasons women are unable to overcome eating disorders.

Beat it by: A dietician, holistic therapist or psychologist's specialised suggestions will aid you to tide over your feelings of loathing and repulsion. After intimately discussing with them, chalk out an improvement plan, and try to maintain it to improve an optimistic personality. Define your personal values which are appropriate for your distinct original self. Only after learning about your internal self, your natural endowment and gifts can you surely uncover the delight and energy to completely develop those gifts, irrespective of what people think or say.

Glucose intolerance - This trigger is physiological. A healthy body not only changes carbohydrates to glucose, but also sustains a blood glucose level of 60-120mg/dl, irrelevant of the intake of glucose by the body. Carbohydrates are transformed to glucose in the glucose intolerant population. An undue amount of the hormone called insulin is secreted by the pancreas in response to this change. Getting rid of the glucose from the blood stream and assisting its entry into the blood cells is the function of insulin. Despite the quantity of consumed carbohydrate, the blood glucose level returns to normal if performed properly. A speedy rise in blood sugar occurs before an over secretion of insulin if this system is inappropriately functioning. As the body cells do not identify the extra insulin, they are powerless to eliminate the glucose from the blood stream. Consequently, the appetite is roused due to the rise in levels of blood insulin, and the person is compelled to eat. The cycle carries on if simple carbohydrates are selected on the diet.

Beat it by: To maintain normal levels of blood glucose, distribute the calories to eat small quantities of food on a frequent basis i.e. every 3 hours. If the time gap between the meal timings is too long, you will be starving or maybe you ate too little at your previous meal. A great deal was eaten at the last meal if one approaches the next meal timing on a full stomach. The possibility to postpone a rise in blood glucose is present in micronutrients of protein and fat combined with carbohydrates. As fat obstructs the value of insulin, protein is favoured, but simple carbohydrates leave the stomach more quickly than complex carbohydrates, thus regulating blood sugar. Fibre is present in complex carbohydrates. This condition can be improved through soluble fibre. There is a chance of superfluous insulin secretion and less appetite stimulation if the blood sugar levels rise slowly. Drinking of water should be increased with a rise in consuming fibre or protein. Nutrients and oxygen are transported to cells and wastes are eliminated by water. Extra water is needed in a high fibre diet for dealing with supplementary roughage and stopping constipation.

Habits - Your daily habits may not be as healthy as they could be and you may not even be aware of some of them. Often, excessive eating, lack of physical activity and stress tips the scales of our otherwise balanced lifestyles. Many people have found that overeating tends to occur in specific places and times, such as in the evening whilst watching TV.

Beat it by: Turning off the TV off and engaging in a hobby that keeps your mind and hands busy. Another solution to stress related overeating is to address the sources of stress. Acknowledge and address feelings of depression, anger or anxiety, and do whatever you can to reduce feelings of stress, like writing a journal, talking with a friend, or exercise.

Lack of energy and feeling tired - You are putting up with so much in your life that this is constantly draining your energy, leaving you feeling tired. "When your energy level is low, you may look for food to pick you up," says Robert E. Thayer, Ph.D, professor of psychology at California State University at Long Beach. Unfortunately, most women reach for calorie laden treats instead of an apple or banana.

Beat it by: Identifying your low energy times of day and substitute them with other activities for eating. Take a 10 minute walk or a water cooler chat break. There are healthier ways of nurturing yourself, such as getting plenty of rest and relaxation, reading a good book, or taking a quiet walk.

Needing Love and Comfort - You turn to food when you're really needing love and comfort. With the pressure of work both at the office aswell as at home women tend to be burned out. All this is acceptable if supported with constant appreciation and love, but lack of appreciation, and discouraging remarks leave women sad and lonely, who tend to turn towards food to find consolation.

Beat it by: Taking out some time for yourself and relaxing, pamper yourself by going out for a facial, manicure or pedicure. If you are male, take out the children to a nearby park where you can walk and relax.

Feeling Overwhelmed - You have got so much that you feel you must do that you find it difficult to take the first step. Pressure of work and deadlines leaves many discouraged, who finally drop out without giving it a try. Take the first step, then the second and third and move on...

Beat it by: Do what can be done, you will be amazed with your own capacity of performance. Reinforce the feeling of achievements in you instead of submitting to the pressure. Emotional eating is sometimes considered well within the range of normal behaviour, however, problems arise when emotional eating becomes excessive and interferes with lifestyle quality and good health. If you feel emotional eating is a problem, it may be wise to work with a counsellor trained in eating disorders

Feeling upset and hurt - You turn to food when someone says or does something that feels upsetting or hurtful to you. Anxieties and emotions can also trigger the desire to eat, and some women eat because they are sad or stressed out or even to celebrate when they are happy.

Beat it by: Going out in the open air and walk, the blast of oxygen will vanquish tiredness and mental exhaustion. Leave your worries behind and be in the moment, look at the birds, be thankful, let go, breathe deeply and relax.

Lack of Willpower - Your attitude is shaped by your thoughts, feelings, and actions, and it's really easy to feel good when the going is good. The key to vibrant energy and a powerful attitude is to MAKE yourself feel good, ESPECIALLY when the going's tough, and you don't feel good, or you don't want to feel good. Willpower is one of the tools you need to employ in order to resist the powerful cravings associated with food. The cravings will attempt to control you, but it is your willpower, determination and self-discipline that you will use to fight back.

Beat it by: developing a strong willpower, and every woman has the capacity to build up or strengthen her willpower by exercising it in times of need. Lifting weights develops muscles, and exercising willpower makes it stronger. Add self discipline in your life to become more aware of how you use your willpower in the course of all your daily activities.

How can negative thoughts keep you fat?

Human beings are always leaning towards a tendency of negative or pessimistic think-ing, and this has a profound effect on our psyche and our lifestyle. Research has shown, from childhood onwards, an average person hears NO about fifty thousand times and YES only eight thousand times. So negative thinking is very deeply ingrained in us. The human brain works in a strange fashion. The brain is likely to connect those thoughts, which you entertain constantly in your mind, with reality and your actions in reality are affected by those thoughts. So if you think negatively then in real life losing weight becomes almost impossible. This kind of pessimistic thinking gradually per-vades your brain and from a conscious thought it sinks down to the level of the subconscious. It becomes a loop you cannot break out of because almost 96% of your behaviour is determined by your subconscious. So these subconscious thoughts deter-mine your day to day activities, and if these thoughts are negative then they can prevent you from losing weight because they induce you to think you can never lose weight.

Usually weight loss programs include a diet and a workout regimen, and these are im-portant, but you must not ignore the mind body connection. Whilst dieting you constantly brood about how terrible the diet is, or while exercising you feel reluctant to perform the exercises, or keep doubting their effectiveness. This way you have no hope of losing much weight in a long term manner. It's impossible to actively love the diet food, the trick is to focus on something else and drive the negative thoughts away from your mind. Discipline your mind and think about things you actually like, as this is the only way to retain an optimistic frame of mind. Your mental activities simply have to correspond with dieting and working out, but you have to back it up with support from your mind, and only then can you hope for success. You have the advantage here, be-cause your mindset is something you CAN control and monitor. It's your choice, think about the wonderful things that accompany loss of weight, think about the positive side and make that choice.

If you focus on what it is you want to achieve by losing weight and think it out before hand then this change to the positive frame of mind will be easy. Create a "wellness vision", what are the benefits of losing weight that appeal to you? Think. Then make them act as an incentive. Make this dream a vivid one, think it out carefully, all its as-pects (physical, mental, aesthetic), should be etched out in your mind. Then dwell on this vision, it will become your pattern of thought automatically. Dieting and exercising are important no doubt, but destroying the built up negativity inside you is no less im-portant. If you choose to switch over to a positive vision and remain committed to this vision, your subconscious will switch over from negative to positive. Repeat this and see whether you cannot lose weight this time, especially if you stay focused and dedi-cated to the cause.

Weight loss hypnosis – (Interrupting negative eating patterns)
Weight loss hypnosis is one of the greatest tools for fighting negative eating patterns which plague our modern society. The reasons behind people developing these negative eating patterns are various and complex, but people need to be made aware of how their habits affect them and how they need to be changed. People must realise the impor-

tance of consuming healthy food and water, which helps in releasing toxic wastes from the body, and how deep breathing encourages metabolism.

The mind also influences the body's state of being to a great extent and people need to keep reinventing themselves continuously in order to empower themselves with healthy habits. You must realise the consequences that the mind bears upon the body as dieting alone is not enough if you are planning to lose those few extra kilos. In order to be successful in your attempt, you must also develop a healthy thought process. The subconscious mind, which has a great impact on our general state of being becomes extremely influential in this case.

One of the fundamental lessons we must learn is to 'Love ourselves' unconditionally.

It is not really selfish on our part if we try and be confident about ourselves, avoiding self pain in the process. Weight loss hypnosis helps us to do so, by replacing the old overeating habits with healthy new ones. It helps us to avoid spicy, sugary and fatty foods and replace them with healthy fruits and vegetables, which in turn ensures a healthy body and mind. It is an old saying after all, that you become what you think and weight loss hypnosis will help you to see yourself in a new light. As it teaches, you must avoid comparing yourself with others, and not to be harsh to yourself if you fail to live up to a certain regimen on a few occasions. In the long run, you just need to cater to your body's actual needs, and not give in to junk foods like sweets and fast foods. Breathing exercises can prove to be extremely handy in these cases as you just need to breathe deeply and rhythmically three times a day for a short time of about 5-10 minutes and the effects can be magical. While inhaling provides you with oxygen, exhaling helps you to eliminate toxins, improving your metabolism rate. You can have a prolonged and healthy life just by developing this breathing habit.

Other than this habit, there is a three step pattern technique which is recognised by hypnotists and dieticians as extremely helpful for losing weight and developing a positive frame of mind. If you ever suffer from attacks of the desire to resort to junk food, or indulge in overeating, you just need to abide by the following steps:

1. Breathe deeply and exhale completely five times;

2. Try and visualise yourself as slim, attractive and healthy. Pay attention to the minutest details of your body, and imagine how good it feels to be looked up to by others;

3. Have a large glass of water, as studies show that many tend to confuse thirst with hunger, and having water always prevents one from overeating.

Weight loss hypnosis can only do its bit by helping you out but you must remember the pros and cons of eating, and try to consciously abide by the three step technique in order to be able to maintain a healthy body and mind.

Body image psychology study

Feelings and emotions keep changing continuously according to our external & internal surroundings. This also affects our perceptive capabilities in the long run. The body image which is sensitive to moods, emotions and the retention of water and weight is thus characterized by a complex blend of its physical and psychological aspects. In 2000, a body image psychology study was carried out by Psychiatric department of University of British Columbia. They published a comparative study of 21 normal women and 21 women suffering from anorexic nervosa. The study proved that the anorexic women were prone to suppressing anger and negative feelings to a great extent. The convoluted psychological issues which lead to a poor body image do not always end up as eating disorders, however these are capable of causing severe damage to our body and mind. You must know that bulimia or anorexia is not caused by poor body image alone, and this can happen to anybody and everybody, and is also capable of affecting school goers and teenagers.

Another comparative study published in 2006 in the Journal of Clinical Child and Adolescent Psychology, was carried out by the University of Melbourne (School of Psychology) in Australia for a span of 16 months. The School of Psychology sought the evaluation of the importance of biological, psychological and social models when it comes to clarifying body image among both normal and overweight boys and girls. The analysis showed that the group of overweight kids mostly suffered from low self esteem as they strived to lose weight. This was brought about chiefly by the unhealthy comparison between the overweight and their peers whose weights were within a normal range. However, the time has come for people to realise that only carrying out body image psychology studies will not help in improving the social conditions, and the health conditions of the individuals concerned. Time has come for us to move on from the why and how, and take adequate steps which will help people deal with their perceptions and cope with eating disorders.

A 12 month study by the University of Washington took matters a step further. The university carried out the study based on the experiences of grade 7 and 10 girls and boys. The study showed that body dissatisfaction and psychological factors which naturally followed it up often influenced social and peer relations. While boys were prone to comparing themselves with muscular idols of their dreams, dissatisfaction among girls was chiefly caused by appearance comparison, and conversations among friends and acquaintances. The study was published by the journal of Developmental Psychology, in 2004.

The neuro-psychology of weight control - winning the brain game

Millions of people have a tough time controlling their weight, as they strive to either maintain a diet regime, or keep thinking that they need to maintain one, until and unless they have already given up trying. In today's world a large section of people are suffering from obesity related problems since they are not aware of the two keys essentials for helping one to stick to high level nutrition and continuously motivate themselves to do so. These keys are carbohydrate management, timing your meals and interactive self hypnosis, which can help you to overcome the yo-yo weight gain syndrome and provide you with a healthy, energized body and a positive frame of mind.

Interactive self hypnosis can help you to win the brain game by helping you to control your subconscious mind, or at least know the way in which it works. Other than interactive self hypnosis, active imagery, visualisation and NLP (neuro-linguistic programming) can also help in controlling weight. The subconscious mind, which is ruled by the right brain, perceives and stores active images which are visual, but actually include all the senses. Specialised self hypnosis education will help you understand how the mind really works and thus enable you to reach your goals easily. The interactive self hypnosis technique is quite simple and thus can be learned and accessed by both children and adults. However, these techniques vary according to clients, since different individuals react in different ways to their surroundings and thus are motivated to respond to specific images and metaphors. The duration of these hypnotic sessions can also vary according to the needs of the individual concerned. These sessions are generally divided into induction, which includes deepening techniques and is then followed up by the metaphoric elements being delivered, and ultimately, the process of emerging.

Self motivation and persistence is stressed upon and given special importance to. This blesses us with better managerial skills in turn, since our society is in a continuous state of flux, due to which quick weight loss programs might not help in the long run. All of these techniques fall under the broad category of neuro-psychology. Interactive self hypnosis increases the focusing abilities of a person, thus enabling them to stick to the necessary regimen and improving their body image and self esteem. Obese people tend to get frightened while trying to come to terms with their new self which emerges having gone through the weight loss program. Fear and anxiety might arise from them not having imagined themselves before in such a way, and interactive self hypnosis sessions help in these cases to release this fear and anxiety. Neuro-psychology helps you to develop a multi faceted approach towards weight loss and thus makes the process more enjoyable for you. It helps you control your mind and body better and helps you taste success in a far more relaxed and easier manner. You can be possessed with a healthy body with a great digestive and metabolic system and an increased level of immunity. In a way, it can be hailed as the ultimate exponent of the Vedic ideal which teaches us the importance of 'Mind over Matter'. Not only are the stress levels decreased, but neuro-psychology of weight control helps us to win the brain game, thus enabling us to lead a healthier and fuller life.

How do you win the brain game?

One's focus of control is what actually determines how the thinking procedure works about one's fate. If one wants to be successful, they have to employ an internal focus of control. The first thing is to identify the internal focus of control, and if one has that, they would think that it is their actions, thoughts, and attitude that control their destiny. They think that the law of attraction has a huge effect on their goals; in other words, if they can see it, they think they can always make it. It is they who control their own fate. If somebody has an external focus of control, they would believe that their destiny is determined by external factors like luck, gods, sun signs, etc. This is not a very good success strategy.

In order to gain success in your venture you must set goals which are achievable. It is always a bad idea to set huge goals which are absurd as failure to achieve goals may set about another fit of pessimism and depression. While losing weight set yourself short term goals and if you achieve them it will fill you with positive energy and by analyzing them you can ascertain the level of success achieved. Your path to your final goal has to be broken up into shorter paths to smaller goals; these should be realistic and achievable and will help you in the long run.

Julian Rotter, a clinical psychologist, claimed that people who have internal focus of control tend to work harder for they believe that it's themselves who would create their own destiny. On the other hand people with external focus of control do not work hard to improve. Research suggested that males have more internal focus of control than women, as do older people, and people belonging to higher professional posts. Though it seems that the internal focus of control is much more desirable and is more successful, often it leads to terrible anxiety, and even depressions. In worst situations, people may start to think that they are incompetent and dumb. On the contrary, often people with external focus of control seem very relaxed, calm, and even happy. These people take life as it comes and at times they feel lucky, and at times unlucky, but they accept whatever they get.

ABC theory and loss of weight
Rational Emotive Behaviour Therapy (REBT) is one of the first behaviour therapies of a cognitive nature, which Albert Ellis came up with in 1953 in order to solve the specific problems of troubled individuals. Through REBT, which is largely based upon the A-B-C theory of personality, Ellis tried to propagate the idea that our emotions are entirely influenced by our beliefs, and not the events which we come across in our lives, as was commonly believed. Ellis was of the opinion that our emotional well-being and our beliefs are directly proportional. It was his belief in his own theory which ultimately became one of the most powerful in the hands of therapists looking to help their patients out by teaching them how to counter their irrational fears and replace them with rational beliefs. REBT suggests that the human mind has the capacity to think both rationally and irrationally. While rationality helps one in being objective in his approach, irrationality distorts, convolutes and misinterprets reality. When it comes to the A-B-C theory mentioned above, A signifies some kind of an event that confronts an individual with a challenge he must pursue in his life. This is called an activating event, and an example of this might be that of a teenager being ditched by his lover.

The B stands for the belief which follows thereafter, affecting the individual's emotions, which is in turn represented by the C. If the individual concerned expects everybody to like him and treat him properly, then his or her behaviour can only be termed as irrational, as he or she is bound to get disillusioned after a point of time. This can only lead to anger or depression. If, on the other hand, the individual is capable of behaving rationally, the disappointing and abrupt end to the relationship will not have a long term effect on him or her. REBT essentially helps in making individuals believe that the emotional consequences are caused not by the activating events, but are influenced in reality by the beliefs of the individuals concerned. To put it simply, it is the thought process which primarily determines how one feels. Thus, while rational people are able to deal almost effortlessly with any obstacle that comes their way, the irrational ones often fail to live up to the challenges of life and suffer frequently from emotional disturbances. As REBT suggests, our self negating irrational beliefs mostly originate from either our own concoctions, or from the viewpoints which other people hold about us during our childhood days. This is however the only thread of connection that REBT maintains with the past. REBT, on the contrary, does not emphasise on understanding one's past at all. The past is unchangeable, and we must work upon replacing our irrational beliefs with rational ones instead, in order to make our present much more pleasant. REBT has done a great deal to spread the word that psychological dysfunction is primarily caused by anxiety and depression, which are only parts of human neuroses. Irrational belief only convolutes one's thought process and drives him deeper and deeper into the world of confusion and continuous self negation as they set themselves unthinkable and almost impossible targets. They slowly develop a habit of continuously assessing them in a negative manner, while they juggle the 'should do', the 'ought to do' and the 'must do' unsuccessfully.

These self effacing beliefs take root in one's mind when he is just a child, and then continue to grow as he keeps revisiting them. This only proves that irrational beliefs can only result in unhealthy emotions, which tend to take a toll on an individual physically aswell at times. According to the A-B-C theory, the consequences of possessing a negative mentality is generally mild, leading to procrastination on many occasions, but in certain scenarios, can also lead to dire circumstances, disrupting and immobilising an individual's general well being.

The irrational beliefs which we have been discussing so far, mostly turn the sufferers into extremists, and these extremist ideals generate the language of the absolute. They more often than not expect themselves to live up to the high expectations of both themselves and others, and everything becomes a 'must do'. What poses the gravest of all problems is that the people concerned are mostly not aware of this unnecessary absolutist behaviour. REBT stresses largely upon mental wellness, and propagates the idea that one can only be mentally stable if he responds positively to any stressful activating event that crosses his path, and the self defeating beliefs are either absent or ignored. This does not however suggest that a healthy person is never going to feel blue, but REBT helps in limiting these derogatory emotions to the bare minimum. REBT equips one with the ability to accept and fight back whatever comes his way. As a result, the individuals who benefit from REBT are made capable of easily accepting their mistakes and quickly learning from them instead of giving in to blaming themselves continuously. Thus, they are able to cherish and enjoy life on a larger scale than the others. Speaking in terms of the A-B-C theory, REBT therapy can be successfully carried out only with a proper understanding of the following steps which are termed as D, E and F. The D symbolizes disputing, one of the primary lessons that the client receives from the therapist so that he can challenge the irrational beliefs. The therapist goes on to logically counter the client's illogical beliefs and makes him seek evidences which might prove that his beliefs are believable.

The counsellor then urges his client to come face to face with the worst possible scenario that might come into being if the client chooses to give up his belief. The therapist also helps the sufferer to believe in his ability to fight back in his day-to-day life, which, having replaced the negative ideals, helps in developing the E, or an effective philosophy, which in turn gives birth to new feelings, or F, which are not derogatory under any circumstances. REBT is not at all interested in the past under any circumstances. Instead, it focuses more upon the present.

The therapeutic procedure might engage the client in carrying out different kinds of homework assigned to him by the counsellor. The homework helps in desensitizing the client by making him come face to face with his worst possible fears and nightmares. The nature of REBT is brief and concise, since it ignores detailed analysis and focuses upon problems which are specific in nature. Another positive aspect of the therapy is that it also teaches the client how to counter all his self negating beliefs in the future, so that, when required, he can properly deal with them without the help of a therapist. REBT, based largely upon the A-B-C theory, helps an individual suffering from self-effacing beliefs to overcome them and enjoy life on a larger and grander scale, as he comes to term with his imperfections, which exist in all of us and are but only a part of life. A proper collaboration between the client and the counsellor treating him with REBT can thus only lead to positive results.

NUTRITION & YOU

"A good way to change somebody's attitude is to change your own."

- George Burns

What is an accurate food requirement for you?

Besides the growling in your stomach, there are several reasons to eat. You may be hungry because there was no nutritional value in your previous meal, you fill a plate to fill an emotional void or you're just plain bored. There is a purpose for food beyond the fact that it tastes good and provides a sensual pleasure for the palate and, if you don't eat, your biological mechanisms will fail, so it is a basic matter of survival. While searching for things that taste good, remember that the functions and mechanisms of your body thrive on whole food nutrition, but unfortunately there is a very large gap between the dietary guidelines and what people actually eat. According to Nicola Reavley, author of Vitamins, Minerals, Supplements and herbs:

- On any one day, an estimated 45% of people don't consume any fruit or juice and 22% don't eat any vegetables. Less than 10% consume the recommended five or more servings of fruits and vegetables;

- Only one third of the population consumes foods from all the food groups on a typical day, with less than 3% consuming foods from all food groups in at least the recommended amount;

- Many diets contain half the recommended amount of magnesium and folic acid. As many as 80% of women who exercise may be iron deficient and the average calcium intake is two thirds of the RDA;

- The average calcium intake of teenage girls resembles that necessary for 3-5 year olds.

With today's hectic schedules, you are lucky to grab three meals a day, much less all the servings of fruits and vegetables that health guidelines recommend. But to fight everything from heart disease to breast cancer to obesity, experts agree that you should eat at least five daily servings of fruits and vegetables, nine being ideal, and in a variety of colours, which reflect different protective nutrients. One serving equals a piece of medium-size fruit; a half cup of fresh, canned, cooked or frozen fruit or vegetables; a quarter cup of dried fruit; or a cup of raw, leafy vegetables.

In case you've been following a low carbohydrate diet and you've done all that is necessary to lose weight, "pumping iron" everyday - the whole works. But you still might not have lost enough weight. In that case, what are the options open to you? All of us have a calorie intake level, reducing which can help us lose weight. There are some "standard" formulas and tables prescribed by nutrition experts when it comes to losing weight. However, these are only theoretically applicable to people of a certain age, height, weight and sex. These methods are hardly suitable for real people, and the only way of figuring out the amount of food required by you for maintaining/ gaining/ losing weight is through experimentation.

Our suggestion for doing so is an effective method, and it doesn't rely greatly on counting calories.

- Decide and set a target weight for yourself, then a time limit within which you want to achieve it.

Avoid using a standard "ideal bodyweight" table, because they usually have a wide range, and muscle mass and bone mass differ from person to person. On the Metropolitan Life Insurance Company's table, the difference between the high end and low end of the ideal weight for a particular height is 30%. You can estimate your target weight by inspecting yourself in the mirror after weighing yourself. It helps to have your health-care provider present who'll have a better idea about judging appropriate body fat. You obviously need to lose weight if you can grab fistfuls of fat on the underside of your upper arms, your thighs, your waist or your belly. Your estimate doesn't have to be absolutely accurate, and you can re-set it as you go along. For instance, if you weigh 200 pounds, you might decide to set your target at 150 pounds. If upon reaching 160 pounds you find that you've lost visible excess fat, then you could choose to stop there. On the other hand, if you still retain some of that excess fat on reaching 150 pounds, then you could reset your target at 145/ 140 pounds before undertaking another visual estimation. The idea is to lose weight gradually, step by step.

- Set a time frame once you've decided on a target weight. Once again, absolute accuracy is not required. Make sure that you don't "crash diet" because it often leads to a "yo-yo" effect, i.e. the metabolism slows down and the excess fat keeps piling up.

If you lose 10 pounds by starving yourself without supplementing it with dietary proteins and exercise, chances are you'll lose 5 pounds of fat and 5 pounds of muscle. If you regain those 10 pounds through carbohydrates, while not exercising, it'll probably be 100% fat. You might even go back to overeating having once reached your target through crash dieting. It's advisable to follow a weight reduction diet which corresponds to what you'll be eating having reached the target. The idea is to stay on the same diet, having achieved your target. This way you don't end up eating excessively and you roughly retain the same diet throughout your life. The trick lies in gradual weight loss i.e. if you're aiming to lose 25 pounds or less, then try losing 1 pound per week, but if you need to lose more, then go for 2 pounds per week. You should consider yourself lucky if you can lose weight rapidly simply by cutting down on carbohydrates. Weigh yourself once a week on the same scale (stripped, if possible) before breakfast, and choose a day, and weigh yourself on that same day each week at the same time of the day. It's not a good idea to weigh yourself more frequently because minor changes in bodyweight occur all the time and you may easily end up misinterpreting them. Losing or gaining a pound in a day is unlikely so stick to your low carbohydrate diet with adequate proteins to supplement it. A simple example explains this: If we assume that you have set yourself the target of losing 1 pound per week. Weigh yourself after a week to see if you've been able to lose that weight and if you have, then continue with your diet in the same way. If you haven't, then the idea is to cut down on the protein at any one meal by a third. For instance, if you have 6 ounces of fish in a meal, then you should cut it down to 4 ounces. You can choose the meal that you want to apply this to, according to your convenience. Weigh yourself again after a week, and if you find that you have lost weight, then you can continue as usual.

If however, you find that you haven't, then reduce the protein intake at another meal by a third. Check your weight again the following week to check for changes. If there hasn't been a difference, then cut down on your protein in the remaining meal. Continue in this manner until you lose weight at the desired target rate. Remember not to add up that amount of protein even if you gradually come to lose weight at the rate of 2/ 3 pounds a week. If you consistently manage to lose a pound a week over a period of several weeks, and your weight has been levelled or balanced, then it's a good time for your doctor to prescribe special insulin resistance lowering agents. An alternate option would be to start cutting down on proteins again, and you can continue with this until you reach your initial target, or until you realise by visual evaluation and estimation that it is no longer necessary for you to lose weight.

To avoid the possibility of protein malnutrition, an average adult weighing, say 150 pounds, would require 9 ounces of protein. This can be adjusted with regard to the ideal bodyweight of an individual. Therefore, ensure that you never reduce your protein intake below this margin. Some experts are of the opinion, that your required protein intake should be twice as much as this, with the idea being to not add back any amount of food once you've attained your target weight. Don't let go just because you've reached your goal, as the trick lies in maintaining this position. Don't immediately put off appetite reducing medications either, therefore wait till your doctor advises you to gradually cut down on them, after about six months or so of achieving your target. If you start binging and eating considerably more than is recommended by your final meal plan, then you might just have to be started on such medication once again. You may well have to stay on such a meal plan for several years, and even if it appears to be difficult at first, it shouldn't take you or your body a long time to get used to it.

Resting metabolic rate
Resting metabolic rate (RMR) is the number of calories it costs for you to keep your heart beating, your lungs breathing, your brain and liver functioning, and all your cells alive and well at complete rest. RMR accounts for approximately 65% of your total daily calorie needs. Of the factors you can control, the main one that affects your RMR is the amount of lean body mass you have. Lean body mass (which includes muscle tissue) is very metabolically active and accounts for 75-80% of your RMR. People who have more muscle on their bodies burn more calories than people who have more fat on their bodies because at rest, one pound of muscle burns up to 70 times more calories a day than a pound of fat. What can you do to keep your metabolism revved up? By regular resistance training 2-3 times per week, older women and older men can recover 10-20 years of loss respectively, with just two months of resistance training three times per week. Resistance training may include any muscle toning exercises, but when it comes to ageing and muscle loss, if you don't use it, you will lose it. In addition to building muscle, which is more metabolically active tissue, very intense exercise sessions can speed up your RMR for several hours after you stop working out. So, people who have more muscle AND are training very hard most days of the week need a lot more calories just to maintain their internal physiological functions at rest.

Are you a fussy eater?

If you are a fussy eater then you can get your intake of fruit and vegetables through a pill. There is, of course, no substitute for a good diet but there are new supplements on the market that come close. (1) Flavonoid complex. (2) Cruciferous-plus. (3) Mixed carotenoid complex, which is not to be taken by smokers (Packer and Colman, 1999). Until you cover all angles and fully prepare, there is no point beginning because you will surely find some excuse not to continue. Perhaps you should even buy the dress or suit that you want to fit into when you have achieved your goal; it all helps with the process. Lasting weight loss, however, isn't just about the body because your mind must be onboard too and throughout the whole process from beginning to end, you have to be honest with yourself. If you want to start with good intentions, you should write a journal about your wishes and desires for where you will be in three months, six months and a year. This book will certainly help you do just that, step by step. According to recent breakthroughs in neuroscience, goal setting, visualisation, positive thinking and the law of attraction are all methods that work. Scientists who have worked with the visual parts of the brain have identified ways to filter out all those things that are unimportant and to call our conscious attention to things that are important involved with reaching our goals.

Imagine the brain is like a computer, waiting for a program to be installed, with the subconscious mind ready to carry out any instructions you give it. Over the years, many of us have picked up negative thoughts with programmed beliefs, habits and automatic behaviour. You may or may not know this but the brain cannot differentiate between real practices and practices that are vividly imagined. Thinking positive and starting with small changes will ensure that your changes become long term, but they should be based on loving yourself and not depriving your body. Even attempting to replace certain late night food choices with an exercise class will help you. Remember though, if this is what you will change, it's important for you to think about how, when, where and with whom you will begin this new exercise class. Whichever way you choose to change, setting a start date is the first phase of putting your plan into motion because having a start date signals the beginning of the new you. Putting it on your calendar, on your mirror, on the fridge or on your PDA will all help you and not let you forget what it is you are trying to accomplish. Think of it as your most important appointment. But remember, this is an appointment for your health and for your new life.

At breakfast time
What you must not do is spike your insulin in the morning with sugary cereal, a bagel or a Danish pastry, because you will be tired and hungry later in the day. Instead, opt for a breakfast that is rich in protein and complex carbohydrates. For example: eggs (not fried) on whole wheat toast. A high fibre, low sugar breakfast is especially crucial because it gradually raises your insulin level, leaving you in good shape for the rest of the day. A recent study compared groups of people who ate egg breakfasts versus groups of people that ate cereal or bagel based breakfasts. The results of the study showed that the egg eaters lost or maintained a healthier bodyweight due to eating fewer calories during the remainder of the day because their appetite was more satisfied, while the cereal/bagel eaters actually gained weight and would have been more prone

to wild blood sugar swings and food cravings. Breakfast (breaking the fast), is the most important meal of the day, and remember that you wouldn't have eaten for 6-8 hours, maybe more, so a healthy breakfast is essential for weight maintenance and mental energy.

At lunch time
Under eating, especially at midday can backfire on you. For example: if you just have a salad at lunch, which includes just a plate of lettuce, this may make you feel full temporarily but you'll also crave those calories later, guaranteed. Eating every 2-3 hours after breakfast will keep your metabolism high, just so long as you are eating sensibly. It's fine to include salads with your meal, but save main course salads for dinner. As for portion control, especially with a whole foods diet (i.e. with vegetables, whole grains and healthy protein), you have the freedom to eat until you're full. On the other hand, flour based products, like pasta and bread or refined foods like white rice, require more attention because these foods affect your blood sugar so keep the portions small (i.e. half a bagel, a cup of whole wheat pasta, etc.). Why not toss tuna and avocado with olive oil and lemon juice and pile it on a slice of whole grain bread?

For an evening meal
Adding protein, like chicken or fish, with plenty of green leafed vegetables will suffice. Overeating, on the other hand, is what got us here in the first place so moderation is key and making more sensible choices is paramount. If you can justify a 'not so good choice' by saying that you will work harder with the exercise, then that is your choice, justification being the operative word. The debate about eating late at night should never be an issue either, so long as the foods are healthy and the quantity is in moderation, but people tend to snack and binge on junk foods.

Snacks in between
Eat plenty of fresh fruits or low fat yoghurts, etc.

As you enjoy the new found energy your new food choices gives you, try and remember that, when it comes to controlling emotions, how you eat is just as important as what you eat. When we look at the whole picture of food regarding stress and mood, we need to include a lot more than just avoiding junk food. Jack Challem, personal nutrition coach and author of The food-mood solution, agrees. "Part of this process comes down to two words, 'be mindful' he said. "People forget this all the time, especially when they're swept up by stress." So, as an example, for your next meal, don't rush your meal in front of the computer. Sit down and savour the tastes with each mouthful and eat more slowly. It takes 20 minutes for the brain to sense fullness, so fast eaters tend to eat more than necessary and, in doing so they quite often wind up with an uncomfortably full belly. Also, take time to pay attention to why you are eating i.e. you could truly be hungry but make sure it's not just because you are lonely, bored or stressed, therefore if you make it a ritual to eat mindfully then you will have a new tool for staying calm and balanced. The key lies in the specific combinations and patterns of the foods you eat. By eating one food before another or with another, you can increase your calorie burn rate by 113% and that's how you can eat 3,500 calories and burn 4,000 or more. Put simply, by eating mostly what you're eating now but re-arranging your food into different combinations and patterns, you'll reach your ideal weight safely in record time. Just by altering and re-arranging your food combinations and patterns, you achieve 24/7 calorie burn to effortlessly and safely melt away excess fat. Food enzymes begin the process of digestion in your stomach, and if there are no food enzymes, your body must produce additional digestive enzymes, which results in fewer metabolic enzymes, but if you eat a diet containing at least 70% of raw foods, you're providing these vital enzymes. Cooking or processing food above 118 degrees Fahrenheit destroys all food enzymes, and if your diet consists mainly of cooked or processed foods, your body's storage of metabolic enzymes will be converted into digestive enzymes. The lack of food enzymes puts a heavier burden on the body to generate adequate enzymes to complete digestion. Eating every 2-3 hours after breakfast will keep the metabolism high, just so long as you are eating sensibly i.e. your snacks are healthy options. For people with weak digestion, it is best to make food combinations as simple as possible. The more you can adhere to a simple mono-diet (i.e. eat one type of food at any one meal), the better your digestive system will cooperate.

Do you know what nutrients your body needs?

Hone in on nutrients most known to boost stress coping ability and try to incorporate more foods containing B vitamins, folate, omega-3 fatty acids and magnesium into your diet. Deficiencies in these nutrients are linked to depression which will, inevitably, lead to more stress. Magnesium, for instance, helps muscles relax, helps you fall asleep and stimulates production of GABA, a neurotransmitter that eases anxiety and nervousness. Stress also prompts your body to excrete more Vitamin C, which is why this vitamin is almost always required as a supplement. So go ahead and add a few extra berries to your morning oatmeal. Antioxidants should also be considered and if you remember us mentioning cortisol, which sets off chain reactions in the body that can damage brain cells and memory, adding these antioxidants will help fight that damage.

Good-mood foods
There's no such thing as a chill pill but certain foods contain body boosting nutrients that will help soothe stressed out nerves, but talk to your doctor about proper dosages if you only take supplements.

Stress soothers
Make the revamp of your daily food choices complete with an emphasis on whole foods (meaning unprocessed and unrefined) and eat them in frequent enough intervals to ward off fatigue and irritability. They'll help your body mellow existing stress and anxiety and set you on the right path for overall health.

How can you re-energise your digestive system?

Recommended for you is a 24-hour cleanse to re-energize the digestive system, which will sharpen your concentration and focus and improve your sleep patterns.
More importantly, it will allow nutrients to be better absorbed into your whole body, which will ultimately provide you with more energy.

1. Drink the juice of one lemon in fresh water during the morning hours;

2. 10-30 minutes later, consume any fruit or vegetable (juiced yourself) or fresh, raw vegetables in boiling water – soup;

3. Water (distilled) should be more than the recommended daily amount. Shoot for approximately ten glasses;

4. Throughout the 24 hours, you may consume any kinds of vegetables prepared as in number two, but the fruit should be one serving and just one kind, no combinations;

5. No salt is to be consumed throughout.

It will vary with each individual, but normally it should take between 1-3 days. You will know how it has gone if you are constantly on the toilet after each meal and if you are not then perhaps you should continue after the 24 hours, but definitely complete the cleanse once or twice a week. "Regardless of the time it takes for your initial cleanse to produce the desired results, going through this cleansing process will become easier and easier in subsequent weeks and your system will become cleaner and healthier as time goes on," says Christopher Guerriero, author of Maximise Your Metabolism. Nutrition tips and diet information from different sources often conflict with each other, so you should always check with your doctor first.

Do you know what your food pyramid looks like?

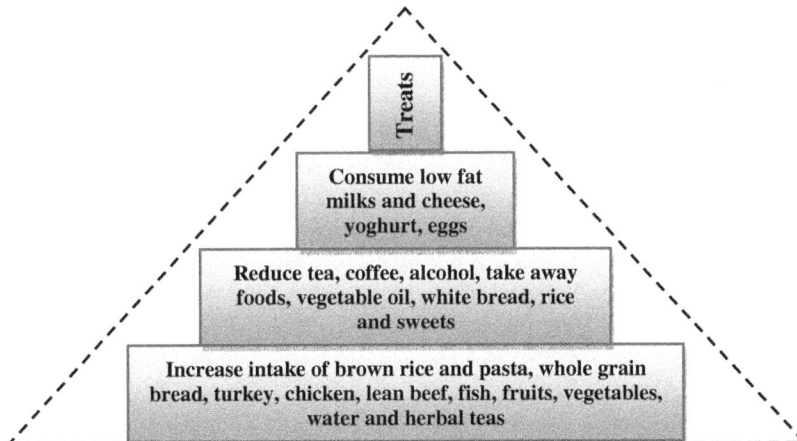

Treats

Consume low fat milks and cheese, yoghurt, eggs

Reduce tea, coffee, alcohol, take away foods, vegetable oil, white bread, rice and sweets

Increase intake of brown rice and pasta, whole grain bread, turkey, chicken, lean beef, fish, fruits, vegetables, water and herbal teas

Balancing your healthy eating pyramid

Before today, you must have seen a 'healthy eating pyramid' which is a diagram that indicates the foods that you should eat more of and vice versa. We have created one of our own especially for you, and you'll discover as you read through the book that eating the right balance of carbohydrates, fats and proteins to include a variety of fresh fruits, vegetables and whole grains will supply your body with the vitamins, minerals, phyto-nutrients and fibre it needs. Sticking to these basic rules is recommended in order to not only weight loss but also to look after your health as a whole. Below is an empty one that you can fill in yourself.

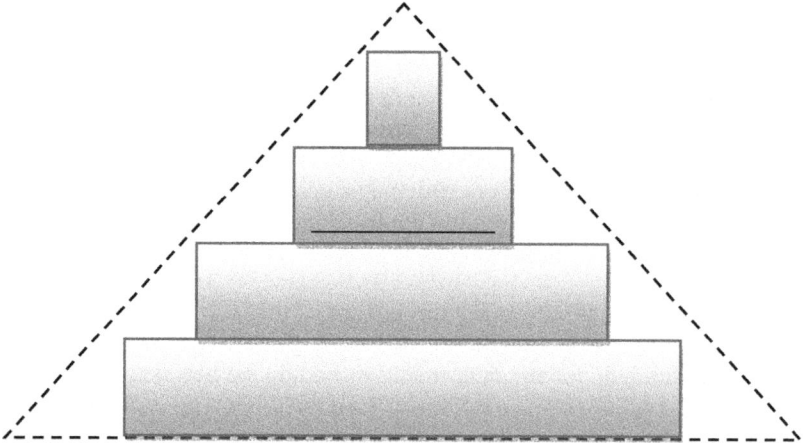

What do you need to know about carbs, proteins and fats?

40 - 50%
The percentage of your daily calories should come from good carbohydrates (beans, whole grains, berries etc). The majority should come from less-refined, unprocessed foods with a low to moderate Glycaemic load (GL). The GL ranks how quickly the body converts food to blood sugar, which can cause greater fluctuations in insulin levels and result in health problems. This will be explained in more detail later in this chapter.

30%
The percentage of your daily calories that should come from healthy fats, mainly mo-nounsaturated (good sources include olive oil, nuts, avocados, etc.) and omega-3s (flaxseeds, fortified eggs, walnuts, or fish, such as salmon and sardines).

20 – 30%
The percentage of your daily calories that should come from healthy lean protein sources, such as chicken, fish, reduced fat dairy products and especially soybeans and soy foods.

As you can see in this example, it is suggesting that you consume a higher percentage of fat than protein. This is because there are a number of healthy fats that our bodies need and this will be reiterated later in the chapter.

Carbohydrates in more detail
The carbohydrate (sugars, starches, and fibres') is the main source of energy for the human body. It is also the fuel that we need so that every cell in our body works effectively and efficiently.

One (1) gram of carbohydrate is equal to four (4) calories.

In our homes we have a carbohydrate choice, which can be compared to the choice we make when we decide which fuel to put in our cars, and with carbohydrates it's either simple or complex. Carbohydrates such as fibres' and starches are known as complex and carbohydrates such as sugars are known as simple, and they are considered simple or complex based upon their chemical structure.When you eat food your digestive system breaks down starches and sugars into glucose that is used to create usable high powered energy for your body. Fibre, however, is not broken down, as it acts as the body's cleanser and the soluble (water absorbent) fibre found in beans and many whole grains may help lower LDL (bad) cholesterol and blood pressure and reduce the risk of heart disease, diabetes, and some cancers. Nature blends the simple and the complex and adds essential micro-nutrients for proper digestion and utilisation of all the carbohydrates, proteins, and fat. Both types contain four calories per gram and both are digested into the bloodstream as glucose, which is then used to fuel our bodies for normal daily activity and exercise. The main differences between simple and complex carbohydrates are explained below:

Simple carbohydrates or simple sugars - The body breaks down and quickly absorbs these foods. This process causes a spike in insulin and, over time, this pattern can cause insulin resistance in some people. But most simple carbohydrates contain refined sugars and very few essential vitamins and minerals. Examples include table sugar, fruit juice, milk, yoghurt, honey, molasses, maple syrup and brown sugar. "The real villain is the food manufacturing industry," says Michael Van Straten, author of Super Energy Detox. He goes on to talk about the sugar in processed foods and how people become accustomed to the 'sugar trap' in foods like:

- Desserts such as ice cream;

- Juices/canned drinks;

- Sugar coated breakfast cereals;

- Biscuits/sweets.

He says that "Once you have acquired a sweet tooth, its not long before every cup of tea or coffee needs three heaped spoons of sugar and every unoccupied moment is filled with a biscuit, a piece of cake or a Danish pastry."

Complex carbohydrates - Complex carbohydrates, however, take longer to digest and don't cause that spike in blood sugar. So insulin is therefore released in a more desirable, gradual manner and is packed with fibre, vitamins and minerals. Examples include vegetables, whole grain breads, oatmeal, legumes, brown rice and whole wheat pasta. A study, published in the American Journal of Clinical Nutrition, showed that people who added whole grains, such as whole oats and whole wheat bread, to their diets lost more weight. Researcher Pauline Koh-Banerjee, ScD, and her colleagues at the Harvard School of Public Health studied 27,000 men aged between 40 and 75 years old and found that the more whole grains they ate, the more weight they lost while dieting. They said that "fibre in the diet may fill people up faster than processed grains and perhaps help to regulate blood sugar levels. Moreover, because of their high fibre and water content, whole grain foods contain fewer calories gram for gram than does the same amount of corresponding refined grain food.

Eating 40 grams of whole grains a day cuts middle age weight gain by as much as 3.5 pounds. All it takes is about 1 cup of oatmeal, or 3/4 cup of brown rice, or several slices of brown bread each day."

Simple carbohydrates & weight loss

As valid research and better information is being presented to the public, people are learning that simple carbohydrate consumption can drastically hinder anyone trying to maintain or lose weight.

CJ Segal-Isaacson, assistant professor at the Albert Einstein School of Medicine, completed a CCARB (Controlled Carbohydrate Assessment Registry Bank) study that examined the physical activity and health patterns of 1,300 people over a three year period. At the one year point in her study, results showed that individuals controlling carbohydrates, eating an adequate amount of protein and increasing their intake of non-starchy, nutrient dense vegetables have consistently maintained weight loss over the last 18 months. In addition, the CCARB study has shown in regression analysis that carbohydrate intake, fibre intake and frequency of workouts were strong predictors of weight change in the reported participants. Of the 34.5 percent of people in her study who have gained over five pounds in the last 18 months, simple carbohydrate consumption, such as added sugar, was the single biggest indicator of the weight gain. It seems clear that consuming adequate protein sources, in addition to non starchy vegetables like dark, leafy greens, and limiting carbohydrate intake can be a viable option for losing or maintaining weight as a long term approach to eating. There is more on protein later in this chapter.

The carbohydrate restricted diet

Studies show that a carbohydrate-restricted diet results in a significant reduction in fat mass and an increase in lean body mass in normal weight men, which may be partially mediated by the reduction in circulating insulin concentrations. There are however, disadvantages to this type of diet and they are as follows:

- For most people, strict low carb diets are difficult to stick to;

- Very low carb diets are often unbalanced and missing many nutrients;

- Very low carb diets may cause low energy levels;

- The initial rapid weight loss on a very low carb diet can be deceiving.

If you remove most of the carbohydrates from your diet for a long period of time, you're setting yourself up for a relapse. What you cannot have you tend to crave, both physiologically and psychologically, therefore, the more you cut the carbs, the easier it is to rebound when you start eating carbs again. You will feel physically tired if carbohydrates are restricted from your diet and you will more than likely become mentally irritable. Your level of energy will be extremely low which, in turn, would equal zero results with your weight loss program. A carbohydrate restricted diet would normally involve the removal of entire food groups, such as fruits and 100% whole natural grains, which is definitely not nutritionally balanced for fibre, phytochemical and micronutrient intake. All of these facts make low carbohydrate diets a poor choice for people who need to get active in order to lose weight. On low carbohydrate diets, water and even lean tissue are much of the initial weight loss. So, if you drop 5-7 lbs in your first week, it will of course sound very impressive, but if one pound is fat, 2-3 pounds is water and 2-3 pounds are muscle, what did you accomplish? Your goal should be fat loss, not 'weight' loss. The few studies that have examined body composition after a carbohydrate restricted diet have reported enhanced fat loss and preservation of lean body mass in obese individuals. A 6 week study conducted by Volek JS, Human Performance Laboratory, Department of Kinesiology, University of Connecticut, reported that fat mass was significantly decreased and approximately 70% of the variability in fat loss on the carbohydrate restricted diet was accounted for by the decrease in insulin concentrations.

Discover the Glycaemic index
The Glycaemic index (GI) is a way of calculating the rate at which carbohydrate foods are digested and converted into sugar by the body. The lower the foods GI, the longer it takes for that food to be converted into sugar. By mixing these foods into a meal, a more even level of blood sugar will be able to be maintained. Using the GI can be a great help in planning a healthy diet that will provide you with a gradual release of energy and in doing so, help you avoid the sugar trap. Weight loss diets may be more effective when dieters seek to reduce Glycaemic load (i.e. the amount their blood glucose rises after a meal) rather than limit fat intake. The findings indicate that a low Glycaemic diet may overcome the body's natural tendency to slow metabolism and turn on hunger cues to 'make up' the missing calories.

Low Glycaemic Load (Low GL) diet
The low Glycaemic load (low GL) diet reduces carbohydrates that are rapidly digested and raise blood sugar and insulin to high levels. Some of the foods include:

- White bread;

- Refined breakfast cereals;

- Concentrated sugars.

Instead, the low Glycaemic load diet emphasises carbohydrates that release sugar more slowly, including whole grains, most fruits, vegetables, nuts, and legumes. Dr. David Ludwig, director of the Optimal Weight for Life (OWL), suggests that "the type of calories consumed, independent of the amount, can alter metabolic rate." He goes on to say, "Almost anyone can lose weight in the short term, very few keep it off in the long term. That's given rise to the notion that the body has a 'set point' and that when you diet, internal mechanisms work to restore your weight to that set point. A low Glycaemic load (GL) diet, may work better with these internal biological responses to create the greatest likelihood of long term weight loss."

Below is an example of the difference between high and low Glycaemic load foods. The figures bracketed in the right hand column dictate slow digestion which means that once eaten, you'll be less hungry later.

OLD FAVORITES *(High Glycaemic load)*	BETTER BETS (Low Glycaemic load)
Breakfast	**Breakfast**
Bagel, white, frozen, 70g *(25)* Instant Cream of Wheat, 250g *(22)* Cornflakes, 30g *(21)* Grapefruit juice, 250g *(11)*	100% whole grain bread, 30g (7) Oatmeal, 250g (13) All-bran cereal, 30g (4) Grapefruit, 120g (3)
Lunch	**Lunch**
Macaroni and cheese, 180g (32) Cranberry-juice cocktail, 250g (24) White rice, 150g (23) Corn chips, 50g (17)	Fettuccini, 180g *(18)* Club soda, 250g *(0)* Brown rice, 150g *(18)* Popcorn, 20g (8)
Dinner	**Dinner**
White spaghetti, 180g (27) Baked russet potatoes, 150g (26) Vanilla cake, frosting, 111g (24) Fanta Orange soft drink, 250g (23)	Whole-wheat spaghetti, 180g *(16)* Baked beans, 150g (7) Banana cake, no sugar, 80g *(16)* Unsweetened apple juice *(12)*

Protein and weight loss

Proteins are molecules made up of amino acids, which the body breaks down and absorbs in order to rebuild and repair tissues. Humans need about 20 amino acids in order to live but our bodies can make most of them on their own. One (1) gram of protein is equal to four (4) calories. As with low carbohydrate diets, there have been studies to show the effect of protein in weight loss. Skov AR from the Research Department of Human Nutrition in Denmark studied the effect on weight loss in obese subjects by the replacement of carbohydrate by protein. It was a study over six months with 65 healthy subjects involved, a mixture of overweight and obese people, 50 of them women and 15 of them men, all aged between 18-55 years.

The weight loss after six months was:

- 5.1 kg in the high carbohydrate group;

- 8.9 kg in the high protein group;

- Fat loss was 4.3 kg and 7.6 kg, respectively;

- No changes occurred in the control group.

Replacement of some dietary carbohydrate by protein improves weight loss and increases the proportion of subjects achieving a clinically relevant weight loss. This study also demonstrates that increasing the proportion of protein to carbohydrate in the diet has positive effects on body composition, blood lipids, glucose homeostasis and satiety during weight loss.

Managing stress with food

Studies show that 90 percent of all illnesses, both mental and physical, are related to stress, therefore, anything you do to dampen that physiological response can help your health. The secret to success is to chill out in stages i.e. grabbing a bit of focused relaxation when you can. Research shows that people who can go somewhere quiet and relax for just 20 minutes, a couple of times a day, are half as likely to be admitted to a hospital. Scientifically, exercise has been shown to reduce levels of stress hormones but remember that any activity that relaxes you counts as a stress reducer. If all else fails, a stress reducing supplement called Holy Basil (available at most health food stores) is a great example of an adaptogen, which helps your body cope with stress and manage cortisol levels. Please note that Holy Basil is not recommended for women who are pregnant or trying to conceive.

Below is a table to assist you:

STRESS FIGHTERS	HELPFUL NUTRIENT	WHY IT HELPS
Avocados, baked potatoes (with skin), bananas, chickpeas, yellow-fin tuna	Vitamin B6	Stress depletes B6, which helps produce serotonin, a calming neurotransmitter.
Clams, milk (fat-free), plain yoghurt (fat-free), salmon, sardines	Vitamin B12	Along with other B vitamins, B12 helps form GABA, a calming neurotransmitter.

STRESS FIGHTERS	HELPFUL NUTRIENT	WHY IT HELPS
Asparagus, chickpeas, lentils, oatmeal, orange juice	Folate (folic acid)	Folic acid helps make dopamine, a neurotransmitter associated with pleasure.
Almonds, amaranth, spinach, sunflower seeds, tofu, wild rice	Magnesium	Stress depletes magnesium, which stimulates the production of GABA and helps make dopamine.
Broccoli, brussel sprouts, orange juice, red and green peppers, strawberries	Vitamin C	Vitamin C boosts your immune system and fights brain cell damage resulting from constant exposure to cortisol.

How to eat your way to a better attitude?

To achieve a constant energy balance and a healthy weight, you must aim to limit your energy intake from total fats and shift fat consumption away from the worst of the saturated fats to unsaturated fats and towards the elimination of trans-fatty acids. You should try to increase your consumption of fruits, vegetables, whole grains and nuts but most of your efforts should be to focus on limiting your intake of free sugars and salt from all sources and ensure that if you have to have salt, it is iodized.

Fill up on fibre
As mentioned previously, incorporate beans, legumes, and whole grains, such as brown rice or quinoa, into your diet. Also, try and add nuts into your diet by sprinkling almonds, hazelnuts or walnuts on cereal or salads or stash them in your desk drawer for a healthy alternative to vending machine rubbish.

Fine tune your fats
Sort out your kitchen and get rid of most saturated fats and all trans-fats by avoiding margarine and anything with hydrogenated oil in it. Replace them with healthier options, such as extra virgin olive oil and flaxseed oil.

Eat more plant & fish based proteins
If you eat a lot of red meat you should attempt to at least substitute it with soy or fish a few times a week because animal proteins contain arachidonic acid, which the body uses to produce pro-inflammatory prostaglandins. Wild salmon, sardines and herring are rich in omega-3 fats and relatively low in the toxin mercury. Attempt to look out for the "Seafood Safe" label or, if in doubt, consider taking a fish-oil supplement.

Attitude to water
Staying hydrated is the best way to:

- Flush out toxins from the body;

- Ease digestion;

- Maintain energy;

- Promote good brain function and all around health.

Think of water as a health boosting beverage and if you want to feel less bloated and leaner, you need to avoid all soda drinks. As for diet sodas with sugar substitutes, they just stimulate a craving for more sweetness. Most people need a coffee in the morning but too much caffeine jacks up your body and confuses your hunger signals. If you work in an office, take in your water and see how better you feel. One week you will have a small bottle on your desk and a month or so later, if not before, you will have a 1.5 litre bottle under your desk...you'll see!

When you feel thirsty, the only liquids you should drink are water or herbal tea because anything caffeinated is a diuretic. Instead, try to drink 100 ounces of water a day. Try filling a 32-ounce container and keep track of how often you have to refill it. Once you've emptied it three times, you've almost hit your target. Aim to empty the first bottle by 10 a.m., the next by 1 p.m., and the last by late afternoon. If regular water bores you, add a slice of lemon or cucumber to your glass (just like at the spa), or try a flavoured, calorie free water.

Attitude to vitamins
Are you getting all your essential nutrients? Believe it or not, 99 out of 100 Americans don't even come close to meeting the minimum standards. Even small vitamin and mineral deficiencies that you have today can lead to big time health problems, such as osteoporosis, tomorrow. Vitamin-C status is inversely related to body mass. Individuals with adequate vitamin-C status oxidize 30% more fat during a moderate exercise bout than individuals with low vitamin-C status. Therefore, vitamin-C depleted individuals may be more resistant to fat mass loss (Johnston, CS, 2005).
Four secrets to vitamin success:

1. Supplements ensure you are covered in case you don't get everything you need from food;

2. If you're female, you probably need calcium and vitamin D;

3. If you're menstruating, you need a multivitamin with iron;

4. If you're vegetarian, you most definitely need iron but a multivitamin alone often won't cut it because iron and calcium can't be given in the same pill as they bind to each other, decreasing absorption.

61

How you take a supplement also matters:

- You must have food in your stomach in order to absorb nutrients, but it's not necessarily as easy as tossing back your pills right after breakfast;

- The compounds in coffee and tea, whether it's regular or decaf coffee or black or herbal tea, will block iron absorption, so don't take a supplement when those are in your stomach;

- Citrus and vitamin-C, on the other hand, aid the absorption of vitamins, so it always helps to take your multivitamin with a little orange or grapefruit juice;

- Line your vitamins up next to your toothbrush, and take them with a small glass of juice before brushing your teeth at bedtime.

Attitude to calories
Our bodies can distinguish one type of calorie from another. We handle fat calories, carbohydrate calories and protein calories differently. Some tend to be stored as fat while others tend to be digested more quickly but knowing the distinction and eating accordingly can help ease blood sugar woes and protect your health.

Attitude to fats
There are still people who believe that fat intake should be kept as low as possible but it's the kind of fats you eat that matters. We hear so much about saturated fat from doctors, nutritionists, fitness professionals, and the media. The fact about saturated fat being bad for us has actually never been proven and, although saturated fat intake does increase your LDL (bad cholesterol), it actually increases your HDL (good cholesterol) even further, hence improving your overall cholesterol ratio. Maybe we need to get our facts straight and figure out who we should be listening to.

Sugar, carbohydrates & Trans fats
Experts agree that these are the big three, the axis of evil that leaves us chubby and cranky. Along with spiking insulin levels and packing on pounds, sugar inflames cells and makes skin more sensitive to sun damage and premature aging. Beyond the way we look and feel there's also our future health to consider. Women who have higher insulin levels from consuming mass amounts of sugar also have a more than 280% higher risk of developing breast cancer. Trans-fats promote inflammation and the production of free radicals that contribute to chronic disorders like dementia, Alzheimer's, arthritis, heart disease, cancer, premature aging, and the list only goes on.

Attitude to cholesterol
All over the world people have become aware of the dangers that cholesterol poses to their health. The greatest risks target the heart, so much so that cholesterol has become synonymous with fatal heart attacks. Of course, this is slightly exaggerated, though in general medical terms, high cholesterol is one of the deadliest afflictions of the modern world.

Attitude to organic foods
Certified organic produce is not essentially healthier than produce that has been grown under non organic conditions and the nutritional content of a particular vegetable does-n't change. But the lack of synthetic, pesticide residues on organically grown produce definitely makes for a safer product.

Attitude to whole grain
There is strong clinical evidence linking the consumption of whole grains to a reduced risk of coronary heart disease (Anderson, 2002). With this disease being the number one cause of death and disability in the USA, in both men and women I'd say that it would be extremely wise to change our attitude towards whole grain foods.

Attitude to Glycaemic load (GL)
Glycaemic load (GL) is a measure of how quickly carbohydrates turn into sugar in your body. When you pulverize starch into flour, it has a huge surface area for enzymes to react on and turns quickly into sugar. High GL foods cause blood sugar to spike and insulin secretion to surge, over time this pattern may lead to insulin resistance, obesity, diabetes and other health problems.

How can you cook & eat healthily at home?

In this day and age we have become accustomed to and have allowed ourselves to be-come limited for time, which is usually because of our poor planning, and because of this, we tend to opt for easy solutions i.e. a drive-thru meal or some form of fast food. If we are at work for lunch, what we should do is prepare something the night before or simply choose a healthier option from all of the choices that are available.

If we can train our mind in this way, it will help solve many issues. When cooking at home, we should always fuel our bodies with foods that are steamed, garden fresh, boiled, baked, roasted, poached, lightly sautéed, or stir-fried but always try and avoid frying at all costs.

Below are some tips to get you on your way:

Snacks, ready to go
You probably have tons of tempting goodies lying around the house and most people feel the need to fill their houses with chocolate and cookies. Psychologically you know they are there and you'll be tempted when you get the slightest bit hungry. To counter-act this you need to make sure that you have a ready to grab alternative in a plastic bag or box i.e. filled with ready washed, peeled and chopped fruit and vegetables that you can pick at or can take with you wherever you go.

Oils
In the kitchen, use extra virgin olive oil for dressings and low heat dishes and use grape seed or expeller pressed organic canola oil for high heat cooking. When it comes to anything generic like vegetable oil, there really is no telling what's inside, so it's best to steer clear of them at all costs.

Salad with everything
Eat a large side salad or a pile of vegetables with every meal and if you add this to the plate first then that just leaves half a plate left for the more calorie filled part of the meal.

Spices
Certain spices, such as ginger, garlic, onion, tumeric and rosemary, have strong anti inflammatory effects so make them an integral part of your diet. Try using ginger, garlic and onion in stir-fries, turmeric in soups and rosemary on roasted vegetables. Chilli is also awesome for weight loss.

Herbs
Throw out all old herbs and make a pledge to use only the freshest herbs, because if you buy fresh herbs they add so much flavour and complexity to food.

Grains
As mentioned before, go for actual grains instead of flour based foods as often as possible, simply because grains tend to have a lower Glycaemic load (GL). This doesn't render bread off limits but try and pay close attention to the texture. For example, if you see big pieces of grain, that's a good sign that it has a lower GL. As for pasta, Italian whole wheat and Japanese soba are highly recommended. Some of the more familiar products that qualify as whole grains under the new definition include oatmeal, popcorn, shredded wheat and brown rice aswell as barley, buckwheat, bulgur, wild rice, whole rye and the more exotic amaranth and quinoa.

Fish
Although it contains an important type of oil, fish is generally low in fat, which makes it a good food for maintaining a healthy weight. The healthiest way to cook fish is to steam, grill, bake and barbecue or microwave it.

However, it is okay to cook fish in a small amount of oil, such as olive, canola or peanut oil. Fish that is deep fried and battered is very high in fat. The same goes for fish cakes, fish fingers and fish served with rich, creamy sauces.

Meat
We now know that protein will fill us up and make us feel more satisfied during and after a meal. Therefore, chicken and turkey would be the healthiest choices and luckily there are endless ways that you can enjoy them in your diet:

- In salad;

- Stir fry;

- Curry;

- Sweet and sour dishes to name but a few.

Know which meats are best

Below is a table of different meat choices and information so you will have more knowledge before you make your next meal.

MEAT	CONTENT	EXTRA INFORMATION	RECOMMENDATIONS
Bacon	Contains about 16g fat per 100g.	Is also very high in salt and usually contains nitrites which, once in the stomach, may form substances linked to cancer. Smoked foods also been implicated as having cancer-inducing potential.	Use bacon in small quantities, and eat only occasionally.
Beef	Contains about 5g of fat per 100g	About half this fat content is monounsaturated fat, similar to the fat found in heart-healthy olive oil.	If you buy minced (ground) beef, make sure it doesn't contain too much fat. The meat facts on beef show that it's fine to include from time-to-time in a healthy diet.
Chicken	Skinless chicken contains around 3g fat per 100g	If you're worried about calories, remove the skin, where most of the fat is found. Chicken is a good source of nutrients	Choose organic whenever you can, both to avoid supporting the battery farming industry and because the flavour is much better.
Duck	Contains 11g fat per 100g meat	Duck contains a lot more saturated fat than either chicken or turkey. It's a good source of iron & zinc.	Eat only occasionally and use in recipes where the skin is removed, such as stir fry's.
Ham	Contains about 3g fat per 100g	Also high in salt. The meat facts on ham don't make very pleasant reading. Packaged ham is often made from off cuts of pork which have been ground, reconstituted with water, starched to bind, then pressed and shaped into 'ham." This kind may be high in fat and additives.	Buy lean ham from a butcher or delicatessen, cut from a joint. Eat only in moderation.
Lamb	Contains around 8g fat per 100g	Lamb is quite fatty, particularly cuts like shoulder. But, as research continues, it's unclear just how harmful saturated fat is to the body.	Lamb is not often reared intensively and, in moderation, is a good addition to a healthy diet.
Offal	Liver and kidneys are lower in fat than meat and are nutritious foods	This is a definite case for buying organic, because the function of both the liver and kidneys is to detoxify the animal's body so they may contain harmful substances if the animal has been intensively reared.	Pregnant women are often advised to avoid liver because of its high vitamin A content, which could be harmful to the fetus.

Pork	Contains about 4g fat per 100g	The vast majority of pigs are intensively farmed so, there's a risk that their meat will contain chemicals such as antibiotics used in factory farming.	Look for organic or 'freedom' meats. These pigs are reared out of doors in communities and have freedom to roam.
Sausages	Contain around 25g fat per 100g	Mass-produced sausages are not only high in fat, they can also contain fillers, additives, lots of salt and mechanically retrieved meat.	Buy sausages from a farmer's market or reputable butcher, who should be using better quality ingredients. Eat only occasionally.
Turkey	Contains around 1g fat per 100g	Star of the meat facts list, turkey is one of the super foods and an excellent lean source of protein. It's also rich in B vitamins and zinc.	Buy organic.
Venison	Contains around 2.5g fat per 100g	Some venison is wild and some is farmed. But even when farmed, deer are seldom raised intensively.	Excellent healthy choice for those who like a robustly flavoured red meat.

If you eat red meat, select leaner cuts, like sirloin steak or filet mignon instead of most steaks, or pot roast instead of hamburgers or meat loaf. No matter what meal you're planning, strike a caloric balance of lean protein, healthy fats and complex carbohydrates. Together, these macro-nutrients stabilise your blood sugar, leaving you less likely to feel famished and desperate for that bag of chips. Your portions should be judged by the size of your fist because the size of your fist is identical to the size of your stomach. Therefore, if you eat more, your stomach has to stretch to consume what you are feeding it. Vegetables and fruits, however, can generally be consumed in large quantities because of their nutritious value. The US National Health and Nutrition Examinations Survey shows that sugar intake makes up 25% of total calories and fat intake approaches 34%, which means that foods that have poor nutritional value make up over half the daily calories.

Believe that eating out can be ok
For many people, restaurant dining is no longer reserved for special occasions, it's more often than not a daily event. However, that food will represent one third of all calories in the average diet. The nutrient content of restaurant meals is extremely difficult to assess and that became apparent when a survey conducted by researchers at New York University found that trained dieticians not only underestimated the calorie content of five restaurant meals by an average of 37%, they also underestimated fat content by 49%. It will not always be possible for you to eat at home so plan ahead. If you are going out for the day with your children to a park, take along a healthy snack, such as an apple with some cheese, or if you are going to a cocktail party, eat before leaving home and avoid the heavy hors d'oeuvres. If you are going to a restaurant and it concerns you by not wanting to ruin your appetite, then carry a small bag of almonds on you. If you have a couple while walking to the restaurant for dinner, then it will prevent you from dipping into the bread and butter.

Your new restaurant tips
If you know what you're doing, it's relatively easy to keep your weight down while eating at restaurants, here are a few suggestions: Come up with a plan. You know what you like but decide what your priorities will be for that meal. If your choice is the fajitas, perhaps you can skip the rice and beans. If it's the cheesecake, order a light dinner, such as shrimp cocktail and salad with dressing on the side. Whatever happens, you should never be afraid to special order with the waiter because the chef will be happy to oblige. For example, if you really have your heart set on the special pasta dish with chicken, sun-dried tomatoes and mushrooms in a spicy cream sauce, consider these changes:

a) Ask the chef to sauté the chicken, tomatoes, and mushrooms in broth rather than oil

or

b) Ask the chef to use just half the cream sauce.

These small requests can result in a dish that is half the calories as the original and all it takes is for you to ask. Most restaurants want to please their customers and are usually willing to satisfy specific requests, such as the five below:

1. Order sauces and salad dressings on the side, or ask for low-calorie dressings;

2. Request salsa, mustard or flavoured vinegars to get fat free flavour;

3. Request half-portions at a reduced price or take home half the meal in a doggie bag;

4. Ask that foods be prepared with olive or canola oil instead of butter, margarine or shortening;

5. Request that foods be boiled or grilled instead of fried.

Eating in restaurants should be a fun experience but you should always stop eating when you are pleasantly full, not when your stomach is cursing at you. If you choose wisely, you can even leave without having to undo the top button of your jeans. If you do crave a dessert, opt for something low fat, like sorbet, fresh berries or fruit.

Gradual changes
*   If you only eat a couple of vegetables daily, add a serving of those at the lunch and the dinner time;

*   Add fruits to your lunch if you don't have much of it otherwise;

*   Be careful while using butter or margarine, and try to reduce its consumption to half;

- Avoid salad dressing as far as possible, or go for fat-free dressings;

- Bring up the consumption of dairy products to 2-3 in a day. For instance, you can drink milk along with your meal, and thus cut down on other beverages. Also, you must prefer low-fat or a fat-free dairy product.

Meat control
- Don't buy meat too often since you will consume it if you have it;

- Meat should be limited to 6 ounces in a day;

- If you are a heavy meat eater, try reducing your consumption gradually;

- Include vegetarian items in your meal instead of meat, wherever possible;

- Increase other nutritious items in your meal aswell, since it will reduce your hunger and desire for meat.

Desserts
- You can use fat-free or low-fat foods for dessert, as they offer good taste and variety aswell. Canned fruit juices can also be used as juices of fresh fruits need very little preparation. Besides, dry fruits can also be preferred since they are easy to carry along;

- Try out some tasty snack ideas like graham crackers, fatless yoghurt, raw vegetables, plain popcorn, etc. They make for very good desserts and can cut down on fats to a great extent as compared to other dessert dishes which you might consume otherwise. In fact, unsalted pretzels make for a great dessert.

Altering selections of foodstuff
Generally we believe that the food we consume is the kind of food that we love. Again it can be rephrased, saying that we are fond of that food as we take it in daily. This re-phrasing is essential as the most precise distinction in the statement generates several potentials for altering a high calorie meal into a trimming meal. The food that I take in on a daily basis appears more attractive and tasty to me in case I suffer from no psychological or emotional distress or shock. Many people have substituted the daily milk by the blue i.e. the non-fat form of milk. At the beginning the blue milk felt dilute aswell as tasteless in comparison to the normal milk and it reminded us of our daily milk. However, after a while we got accustomed with the blue type to such an extent that the normal milk started feeling too concentrated. This shows that we start liking that which we consume every day. Here is a fundamental rule that lies beneath the triumph of the weight shedding schemes. Foodstuff rich in fibre but lacking in calories is taken in for months. It is noticed that at the end of the specific period the taste buds have become accustomed to this food and they start tasting good. You can follow this Add-A-carrot scheme at your own place and you will notice that your tastes have definitely altered. In case you want to be fond of more nutritious food then make them a part of your meals.

After you make a meal, split it into seven or more containers and keep warming it all through the following week. You can also apply the same technique to beans, soup, or any other nutritious food that you wish to be an integral aspect of your meal. However, if in your childhood you have been compelled to eat them, then you might have to work harder.

Food training: Concentrate absolutely on the food that you eat in your following meals i.e. think only of the taste, the smell, the very deed of eating, emotions and other things related to the meal. This will assist you in two manners: (1) it will get your attention to the present act and thus allow you to be satisfied with whatever you are taking in (2) it might also keep your weight in check as in most weight loss schemes one significant factor is that you need to be conscious of your entire meal process. When a parent wishes to alter the food habits of their children, then they should provide the child with some incentive after every spoon of food they gulp. The gifts could be a lengthier story time or that they can watch TV for longer than they generally do or anything that you choose. Gradually your child will love and start appreciating the food that is given to him or her every day.

Success Tip - Flavour in place of fat: One of the recurrent patterns seen in and out of tradition is that we generally eat food that are very rich in calories, but again when we need to shed off the extra fat , we are discontent with the kind of foodstuff that we are expected to eat. The only solution is to add a bit of flavour to our fat free food so that we start liking them. Just plain green beans do indeed taste bland, but if I add garlic salt and lemon juice in place of butter then I do cook up a delicious meal, thus I feel content too. You can have your own ideas to make your fat free food taste good i.e. if you are fond of garlic aswell as onion, then you can add garlic powder aswell as onion flakes in three of your vegetable dishes in the following week. Be innovative and repeat these ideas in cycles so as to like the food you are eating. The other add-ons that you can use are spices, lemon juice, low salt soy sauce, poppy seeds, salsa or any other Flavour that you like.

Not fearing the fats
A healthy perspective will state a reduction in the fat intake of the western world, but low levels can be alarming. For providing essential fatty acids and fat soluble vitamins and the latter's absorption, fatty acids are essential. The body cannot produce good fats like omega-3 fatty acids, needed for brain functioning and development of children, possibly keeping heart disease and arthritis away, on its own. A low fat diet will help in weight loss because of a consumption of reduced calories as a gram of fat is equivalent to nine calories. Dietary fat plays a role in weight loss and maintenance as indicated by present scientific evidence like the CARMEN study completed at the Nutrition and Toxicology Research Institute in the Netherlands by Saris WH, who examined the long-term effects of alterations in dietary carbohydrate/fat ratio and simple versus complex carbohydrates. The study was extended over six (6) months among 398 moderately obese adults divided into two (2) main groups:

1. A low fat, high simple carbohydrate group;
2. A low fat, high complex carbohydrate group.

The findings suggested modest but significant loss of bodyweight and fatness is the result of lessening fat intake. Substantial differences in weight were not suggested by increasing either simple or complex carbohydrates. The significance of this dietary change and possible effect on obesity's public implications are stressed by these findings.

What to look for on food labels?

In the grocery store is where your secret to success begins, especially if you eat at home on a regular basis. If you do, you must read package labels. It would be wise to study the ingredients of foods advertised as:

- Low / non fat;

- Fat free;

- High protein;

- Low cholesterol / carbohydrates etc;

- Reduced sugar. Pass on any food that names sugar as one of its first three ingredients, even if its sucrose, high fructose corn syrup, brown sugar, or honey as it's all sugar.

Dietary Components - Labels on foods have changed so much over the years but now the FDA and administrations like it have taken on the task of making the most sweeping changes to food labelling in a generation. Susan Thom, a registered dietician of Parma in Ohio, knows how important it is for people to know the number of calories from fat they eat each day. She states that "you need to limit fat consumption to 30 percent or less of total daily calories." But in the past, obtaining that information from the food label has required some mathematical skill, namely, multiplying the total grams (g) of fat in a serving by nine since 1g of fat contains nine calories. She also says that, "it does take time, but if you want to feed yourself well, you have to look at the label." For millions of people who seek to restrict their fat intake to recommended levels, a new dietary component has been added to the food label - 'calories from fat.'

Trans Fat

70

Whatever you do when you are out shopping and checking labels, you must reject anything with trans-fats, which may be listed as partially hydrogenated vegetable oils. Remember to crunch the numbers on the labels. If you buy a product like crackers and they claim to have zero trans-fats in them, look closer at the label. You may find that it has less than half a gram per serving, which might be listed as three crackers. Of course, when you eat three servings (i.e. nine crackers), you're getting too many trans-fats in your system.

In this case, the ingredient list reveals more than the nutrition label. A product can say zero trans-fats and still have a small percentage. How so? The FDA allows for up to half a gram of trans-fat under the "zero" label. The Institute of Medicine, however, maintains that there's no safe minimum level of trans-fat. Look out for ingredients, such as shortening or partially hydrogenated oil, to tip you off that the food contains some trans-fat. If a food has just one gram or more of combined saturated and trans-fats per 100 calories, you must put it back and should aim to want to get your trans-fat consumption down to zero.

Colour of food
You should always consider a foods colour, especially in breads, rice and pasta made from whole grains, which are often brown. These are definitely what you need as they are digested more slowly than refined white ones. As you have read previously, the body processes white bread, rice and pasta as sugar almost immediately, causing insulin spikes. So if you endeavour (over a period of time) to replace every white food you eat with something brown, then you will definitely notice the difference.

Soy
We hear a lot about the benefits of soy but, as with most things, moderation in this particular case is paramount as you can definitely eat too much soy and the type of soy you eat matters greatly. It's desirable to eat moderate, regular portions of fermented soy foods, like Miso and tempeh, traditional foods whose health benefits have been shown in Asian population studies. But, when it comes to highly refined soy products, such as fractionated soy foods, Tofu, soy protein isolate or added soy isoflavones found in certain protein powders and energy bars, there's no comparable evidence for health benefits. Soy isoflavones may carry risks associated with thyroid dysfunction so it's best to stay away from them.

Organic labelling
Organic junk food is still junk food. Some foods sound healthier but with all the sugar and oil, they are just a disguised version of the same thing minus the pesticides. To be 100% sure, read the labels first and of course use common sense.

Whole grain labels
When you buy products labelled "whole grain," you may assume you're getting a healthy dose of fibre, which helps keep your digestive system running smoothly and reduces your risk of numerous diseases. But like "organic," terms like "whole grain" can be misleading on packaged foods so always check the fibre content. The FDA states that whole grain foods should contain the three key ingredients of cereal grains:

- Bran - the fibre filled outer part of the kernel;

- Endosperm - the inner part and usually all that is left in most processed grains;

- The germ - the heart of the grain kernel.

Plus, these three ingredients need to be present in the same relative proportion as they exist naturally, a way to be sure that manufacturers do not add back small amounts of each ingredient to highly processed food and then call it whole grain. While these guidelines are aimed at food companies, Barbara Schneeman, director of the FDA's Centre for Food Safety and Applied Nutrition said "it's also very important for consumers to have consistent and uniform terminology for what consists of a whole grain."

Shopping list for slow burners
We have listed some foods below and overleaf for you so that you can use them as additions to your shopping list.

This list is by no means inclusive of all the ones you need in order to speed up your metabolism, but just try them out for yourself.

ANIMAL PROTEIN	VEGETABLES	FRUITS
HOOFED	**FIBROUS** **3 - 5 A DAY**	**2 – 4 A DAY**
Beef (lean)	Bean sprouts	Apple
POULTRY	Beetroot	Apricot
Chicken	Broccoli	Banana
Eggs	Brussels	Cantaloupe
Turkey	Cabbage	Cherry
DAIRY	Carrots	Grapefruit
Low fat cheese	Celery	Honeydew melon
Low fat milk	Cucumbers	Orange
Low fat yoghurt	Green beans	Peach
SEAFOOD	Kale	Pear
Catfish	Lettuce	Plum
Cod	Okra	
Flounder	Onions	
Haddock	Peppers	
Perch	Spinach	
Scrod	**STARCHY**	
Sole	Potato	
Swordfish	Squash	
Tuna	Yam	
Turbot		

VEGETABLE PROTEIN	GRAINS & GRAIN PRODUCTS	FATS & OILS
Miso	Brown rice	Olive oil
Tempeh	Kasha	Sesame oil
	Oatmeal	Canola oil
	Berries	Quinoa
		Butter
BEVERAGES		
Water (approx. 2L or x8 glasses)	Herbal or any flavoured tea	Any blended vegetable juice or fruit juice using the above foods

Which beverages should you choose?

The beverages listed at the bottom of the shopping list (above) are your best bet for weight loss and you should try as much as you can to avoid the following:

Slim fast shakes
Which are full of:

- Many chemicals;

- Hydrogenated oils;

- Fructose corn syrup.

Attempt to blend your own using skimmed milk, egg and any fruit you like, especially fresh or frozen berries.

Soda (fizzy drinks)
Soda is a carbonated cocktail full of nasty chemicals and gut fattening high fructose corn syrup. This is the most evil thing you can put in your body and causes a myriad of health problems.

Diet sodas are full of artificial sweeteners which:

- Create a negative hormonal response;

- Increase fat storing hormones;

- Increase cravings for sweets and refined carbohydrates.

Cost
The manufacturers of junk foods would love for you to think that healthier options are more expensive but if you shop wisely, you'll see that some of the healthier food op-

tions don't cost that much more, if at all. In general, the less packaging, the less you'll pay and you will find that if you venture into a health food store and compare, you will be surprised by how inexpensive the foods are. Bargains are also found at farmers markets because there's no middle man and of course a reduced transport cost. Most processed foods are downright cheap but you must consider why?

The reason is because many processed foods are made with government subsidised ingredients, like corn oil and high fructose corn syrup. Even if they're inexpensive on the shelves, they're no bargain health wise. According to OZ Garcia, author of The Balance, "Certain foods speed up a sluggish metabolism, give you more energy and build up your resistance to diseases to which you may otherwise be prone."

IT'S YOUR BODY

"A march of a thousand kilometres begins with a single step."

- Chairman Mao

Do you allow your body to function as it should?

If you believe that calorie restriction alone can help you achieve all that you desire for long lasting results, then let me put out your fire. This belief alone is a short sighted and incomplete approach to a complex problem. What is required is a complete change in lifestyle habits to achieve better health, better body composition and results that last.

Before this subject is addressed fully, you must ask yourself the following questions:

1. How active was I when I was younger?

2. What activities have I tried in the past?

3. What did I enjoy doing the most?

4. How active am I now and how can I step it up a gear?

Once you have answered those questions, then you will have some idea of why we say that you must move to get to where you want to get to. But, before we do that, maybe we should take a look at how society has changed over the years and, more importantly, how we have let society rule us. We must acknowledge that at present, the majority of us own a car whereas people never used to go anywhere before without walking, cycling or running to wherever they wanted to go. At work and at home we have computers where we can tend to spend many minutes or hours just sitting there. We settle for texting, phoning and generally communicating with friends and family that possibly live just around the corner or within walking or cycling distance.

At school level and with children is where the education needs to start, instead of them sitting in front of the TV or Play Station for hours on end exercising their wrists or backsides, they should be playing all sorts of games and sports close by the house with their friends. What happened to climbing trees (safely), making play dens, tree houses or just simply playing hop scotch or skip in the back garden….where did all that go? There seems to be less value for physical education these days especially during school hours, let alone after school programs. So what chance do we have in moving our way to a healthier future with our families?

Different types and amounts of physical activity are required for different health outcomes, take a look at the difference between activity and inactivity:

Physical activity is defined as any bodily movement produced by skeletal muscles that require energy expenditure. Michael Van Straten, author of Super Radiance Detox, suggests that "with weight bearing exercises, you can prevent osteoporosis, a life threatening and ageing disease." He also states that "one in three women and one in twelve men will develop osteoporosis and tragically, it's happening in younger and younger people."

Physical inactivity is of course a lack of physical activity but it is an independent risk factor for chronic diseases. It is estimated to cause approximately 1.9 million deaths globally.

Physical activity and health is a key determinant of energy expenditure and thus is fundamental to energy balance and weight control, it also:

- Reduces the risk of coronary heart disease and stroke;

- Reduces risk of Type II diabetes;

- Reduces the risk of colon cancer and breast cancer among women.

How can excess body fat affect your body?

An overweight person having increased levels of inflammation is a known scientific fact. Today, the tracing of a part of this inflammation to the fat itself is believed by scientists. Fat cells churn out low grade systemic inflammation proteins called cyto-kines in overweight people. Pro-inflammatory omega-6s are found a lot in refined vegetable oils like corn and safflower. Adding that low-level inflammation may contribute to disease, location is important for excess body fat, and the fat surrounding our abdomen is the greatest source of inflammation. Large quantities of anti-inflammatory flavonoid compounds are found in cherries, blueberries and blackberries. Astrup A. and colleagues completed a study at the Research Department of Human Nutrition & LMC in Denmark. The role of dietary fat in body fatness was studied by them.

The study concluded that:

- Fewer calories in a low fat diet, with high proteins and fibre rich carbohydrates (primarily from different vegetables, fruits and whole grains) are more satisfying than fatty foods;

- The most beneficial effect on blood lipids and levels of blood pressure are seen in this diet composition providing good sources of vitamins, minerals, trace elements and fibre.

In people of normal weight, reducing dietary fat without restricting total energy intake prevents weight gain, and this same diet produces a weight loss in overweight subjects which is of course highly significant for public health.

How do you get more energy before, during & after exercise?

- Before - If you're exercising for less than an hour, a bagel, toast, plain pasta, a banana or crackers are all good carbohydrate choices one to two hrs prior to exercise;

- During – Sports drinks, bananas or sports bars or just plain water are good options;

- After – 1-2 hours after exercising your priorities are carbohydrates, and to replenish the fluids lost during your workout.

Research shows that it makes no difference in performance whether you drink your carbohydrates or eat them. Drink at least one glass of water before and after your workout and every 10 to 15 minutes during your workout to replace fluid lost in perspiration.

You will want a higher intake of minerals (particularly electrolytes) and water soluble vitamins (vitamin C and all of the B vitamins) since you will be using them up and sweating them out at an accelerated rate.

As a side note, instead of drinking high sugar sports beverages you might want to consider just adding liquid trace minerals to your water.

Exercise your mind & body:

1. Exercise increases your metabolism;

2. Exercise creates a caloric deficit without triggering starvation mode;

3. Exercise helps you sleep better and manage stress better;

4. Exercise (strength training) tells your body to 'keep the muscle' while dieting causes muscle loss;

5. Exercise increases bone density;

6. Exercise helps prevent diabetes, controls blood sugar and improves insulin sensitivity;

7. Exercise improves cardiovascular health;

8. Exercise improves mood, helps relieve depression and increases self esteem;

9. Exercise increases mobility and quality of life as you get older;

10. Exercise helps you keep the weight off long term.

How can you prevent injuries?

Most injuries occur to ligaments, tendons and muscles, with only about 5% of sports injuries involving broken bones. Most frequent sports injuries are sprains (injuries to ligaments) and strains (injuries to muscles) caused when an abnormal stress is placed on tendons, joints, bones and muscle.

Ways to reduce injury:

- Wear the right gear - Wear comfortable sports clothing and appropriate footwear and prevent heat injury by wearing lighter clothing;

- Increase flexibility - Stretching exercises before and after exercise can increase flexibility;

- Strengthen muscles - Adding resistance exercises to your workouts strengthens the muscles;

- Use the proper technique - Good form should be reinforced during the initial stages;

- Take breaks - Certain rest periods can reduce injuries and prevent heat illness;

- Stop your workout - If there is pain;

- Avoid heat injury - Drink plenty of fluids before, during and after exercise, decrease or stop during high heat/humidity periods.

Post injury
The moment you realise you've injured yourself, you'll need to take some steps to secure a full recovery later on. One of the most effective methods of treatment is R.I.C.E.R.

Rest
This will help to slow down the blood flow to that area of the body and prevent any further damage;

Ice
The most common recommendation is to apply ice for 20 minutes every two hours for the first 48-72 hrs;

Compression
Helps reduce bleeding and swelling around the injured area and provides support for the injury. A wide, firm, elastic compression bandage can be used;

Elevation
Raise the injured area above the level of the heart at all possible times, which will further help to reduce the bleeding and swelling;

Referral
If the injury is severe enough, it's important that you consult a professional physical therapist or qualified sports doctor for a more accurate diagnosis and they'll be able to tell you the full extent of injury, and assist if you have additional questions or concerns.

How your posture can be the making of you
To excel in any physical activity and reap maximum benefits you need to have a solid foundation built on perfect form. People definitely take posture for granted, pretty much like breathing, and they rarely consider it when exercising. Bad posture and incorrect technique can cause imbalances in your muscles, which in time leads to injury. You can tell so much from a person when you look at their posture, as it can affect a person's presence, stature, and more importantly their confidence. Here's exactly what it entails:

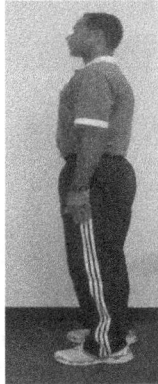

Head up, chest out, shoulders and arms relaxed.

Natural stance instructions:

1. Stand with your feet side by side about shoulder width apart;

2. Raise up on the balls of your feet;

3. Now gradually lower your heels until they just barely touch the floor;

4. Push your sternum out slightly;

5. Tuck your chin in a little;

6. This is going to feel a little weird, lean forward ever so slightly from your hips.

81

Breathe your way to health

As with posture, breathing during any form of exercise is often taken for granted, we obviously breathe all the time but often underestimate how much the way we breathe helps during our exercise routines. Many people make the mistake of unconsciously holding their breath when doing a strenuous activity, but this in turn causes unwanted tension in the muscles, making the activity that much harder. Breathing properly promotes blood flow and increases the delivery of oxygen and nutrients to your muscles, which charges the whole body with more energy. Breathing is the most important physical principle to refine before an exercise or movement.

The following points should be considered;

- Relax the shoulders when breathing;

- Never hold your breathe;

- Breathe in through the nose for five seconds and out through the nose or mouth for five seconds.

What do you need to do to prepare your body?

Your muscles, ligaments and tendons have to be warmed up so that they are less likely to be injured. You should try and pick a warm up activity or choose movements which call into action the muscles that you will be using during your workout.

The following should be included to ensure an effective and complete warm up:

Pre-exercise warm up

This phase of the warm up consists of 5 to 15 minutes of light physical activity and the aim is to elevate the heart and respiratory rate, increase blood flow and increase muscle temperature. If you are going to complete an upper body workout, then start off at the top by gently moving your shoulders, then gently move your head from side to side and up and down. Then work your way down to the shoulders again with gentle arm circling, forwards and back and side to side. Mobilise all the joints of the upper body in all ways until your muscles feel warm and your joints move more freely prior to the stretch phase. If you are going for a walk or a run then you should be mobilising your lower body prior to the stretch. Move the hips, knees and ankles forwards and back and side to side to warm the muscles. Jogging forwards and back, side to side, raising the heels to your backside and knees to your chest are all different ways you can raise your heart rate and prepare yourself for the stretching phase.

Static stretching

The next 5 to 15 minutes of gentle static stretching should be used to gradually lengthen all the major muscle groups and associated tendons of the body, which increases your range of movement. This helps you move freely without restriction or injury occurring. The easiest way to remember how to breathe during a stretch is to exhale as you are moving into the stretch and inhale as you return to your original position.

Breathing slowly and easily also helps to relax your muscles, which makes stretching easier and more beneficial. Check with a physician before completing any of the following: (Think about posture with ALL stretches. The head, shoulders and hips need to be aligned at all times).

Light stretches for walking, jogging, running and all lower body exercises:

1. Gluteus Maximus

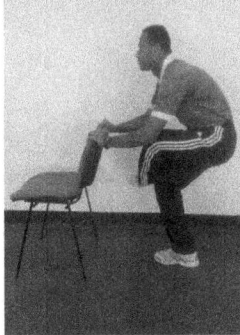

Buttocks and outer hip - Place the ankle just above the knee of the supporting leg, which should now be bent, and move your hips back and use support for balance if required.

2. Hamstrings

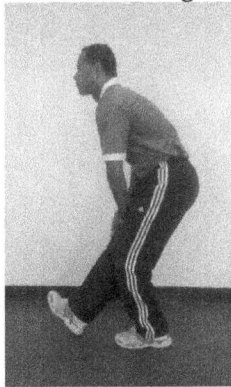

Back of the leg - Bend the back leg at the knee, lean forward with your upper body and feel the stretch more by raising the toe of the straight leg.

3. Quadriceps

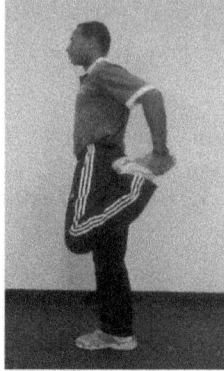

Front of the leg - Lift the heel of the bent leg towards your buttocks whilst keeping the thighs and knees close together.

4. Hip Flexors

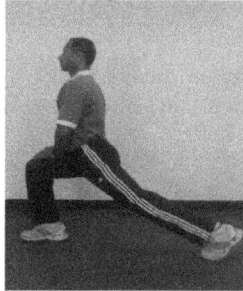

Front of the hip - Bend the front leg to approximately 90 degrees, the rear leg needs to be bent at the knee to feel the stretch at the front part of the thigh of the rear leg.

5. Calf

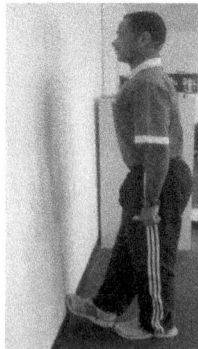

Back of the lower leg - Raise the toe of the front leg and use your bodyweight to increase the stretch of the calf of the straight leg.

Light stretches for upper body exercises:

6. Triceps

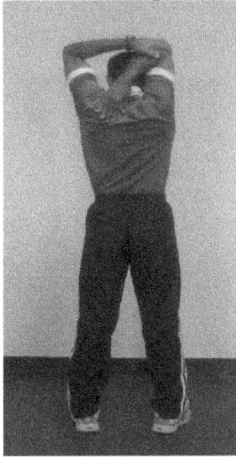

Rear View

Back of the arms
Bend the elbow of the arm that is over your head and push downwards on the elbow with the opposite arm.

7. Posterior deltoid

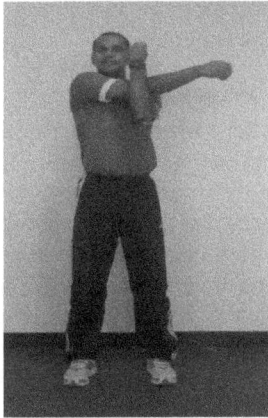

Back of shoulders
Pull the straight arm across the chest by grasping just above the elbow with the opposite arm.

8. Anterior deltoid & pectorals

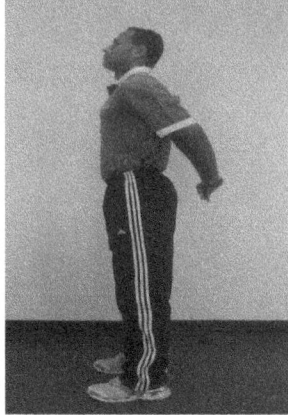

Front of the shoulders and chest
Expand your chest and pull your shoulders back while pulling your clasped hands away from your lower body.

Prior to commencing your exercise program, you need to raise the heart rate even more. After the stretches have been completed, repeat all the movements that you did in the warm up phase but much quicker so that you can raise the heart rate and temperature of the muscles prior to the exercise program.

Post exercise cool down
The reasons why you stretch after exercise are very different to warming up, but are just as important and very necessary for a number of reasons. Any strenuous activity, particularly weight lifting, causes a small amount of damage to the muscle and associated soft tissues. These small rips and tears are what force the muscles to grow when they begin the process of repairing themselves. Damaged tissue is replaced by stronger tissue, which, for up to 48 hours after exercising, often causes soreness. This is called DOMS or Delayed Onset Muscle Soreness. On completion of your workout your muscles are warm and elastic, and the post workout stretching session affords you a second chance to increase your flexibility and range of motion, particularly around your joints. Regardless of the type of activity you should stretch all major muscle groups, including your abdominals and lower back.

Does your body get enough rest?

A lack of zzz's impairs your body's ability to heal itself and lowers brain function. Studies have shown that a person who gets only five hours of sleep can exhibit the motor skills of someone who has drank two alcoholic beverages. Staying up late also screws up cortisol levels, putting you more at risk for diabetes and obesity.

Secrets to success:

- Try to hit the sack by 10 p.m. and get eight hours of rest, and if you go to bed at 10 and wake up by 6, your body will get its optimal levels of healthy hormone fluctuations. If you can't make it to bed by 10, then go to bed by midnight and get up at 8;

- If you're a night owl, naturally train your body by going to bed 15 minutes earlier each week. If you toss and turn once you're under the covers, don't self-medicate with over the counter remedies as they can leave you with a morning hangover effect;

- Dim the lights a half an hour before bedtime and turn down the heat, as low light signals your brain that it's time to sleep and cooler air promotes the small body temperature drop that occurs when you sleep;

- If all else fails and you don't get your eight hours, make it up by napping. A 15 minute nap can make you feel infinitely better, although anything longer than about 20 minutes can be too much of a good thing, as if it's too long or too late in the day it can interfere with your night time sleep.

Melatonin, which is our natural sleep hormone, spikes between midnight and 1a.m., so you don't really want to be awake then. It's a very powerful antioxidant and anti-inflammatory and it decreases the amount of oestrogen your body produces and it stimulates your immune system.

YOUR LIFESTYLE

"Success is not the result of spontaneous combustion, you have got to set yourself on fire for it."

- Anonymous

How easy is it to walk away from your past & into your future?

To get you started with movement, let us take a look at walking and just a few of its advantages. A walk may be just the thing you need to get you through your day. It can set the stage for inspired thinking and major mental breakthroughs because when you walk, you stimulate portions of the brain in the right and left hemispheres, giving you access to more areas of your brain than when you're sitting still. A million years of evolution have equipped our bodies to operate in an optimal way when we're walking and its part of our body's normal restorative process. Walking not only lowers your stress levels, it allows you to sleep better, improve your mood and of course it assists your diet regarding weight loss.

A few other advantages of walking are:

1. It is simple;

2. It is cost effective;

3. It is enjoyable;

4. You can walk anywhere;

5. You can walk at anytime;

6. It is low impact;

7. It is easy on your joints;

8. It is easy to fit into your day.

Technique for walking
Believe it or not, there is a technique for walking as there is for all activities of fitness, but it mainly correlates to maintaining the correct posture.

Lift your head
A jutting head or chin can throw your neck and spine out of alignment, which in turn can cause strain. Therefore, you should lengthen the spine and the back of your neck to bring your shoulders to the proper position and allow your spine to unfurl. These pointers should help your body find its natural alignment.

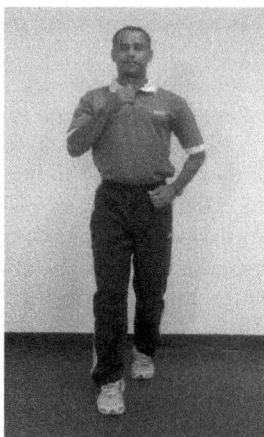

Engage your abdominals

A weak core, which puts excess pressure on the discs between your vertebrae, causes compression in the spine that can result in disc degeneration over time. Therefore, you should gently draw your navel in toward your spine to strengthen and stabilise your core muscles. All of these pointers will help tone abdominals, reduce pressure on your discs and will ultimately safeguard you against back injury. Better alignment of the pelvis, spine and rib cage protects your knees and lets your skeleton support your body more efficiently.

Don't squeeze

Overactive glutes work overtime even when they don't need to and this is often an un-conscious attempt to stabilise the body. Clenched buttocks push the thigh bones forward, constricting the hips and lower back. Therefore, you should release the glutes as you walk and let your hips drift back slightly so they can sway naturally. All of these pointers will help reduce lower back strain and reduce tension. Plus, allow your abs to engage and stabilise the body rather than rely on your glutes to do the work.

Short stride

Over striding, which causes your leg muscles to work too hard, forces the knee into hyperextension, which can degrade the joint over time. Focus your energy forward and keep hips, knees and ankles in line by taking narrow, straight steps.

Progressive

Once the correct technique and posture have been mastered, then the pace and/or the distance can be gradually increased for more rapid results. Once your heart rate is in-creased then the body can become more conditioned. Working out too hard though, may boost inflammation levels rather than reduce them and, while some muscle sore-ness is warranted, if you're feeling exhausted or overly achy, rest a day before hitting the exercise again. All the walking in the world won't do you any good if you're tweak-ing your knee, jostling your spine or overtaxing your tight muscles.

While walking, the breathing should be deep, which will ensure that your lungs are being filled in a comfortable manner (during inhalation) and the exhalation should not be forced too much. The best advice is to breathe however you feel comfortable, although it is advised to try and breathe in through the nose and out through the mouth. Once you have been walking for some time and your body has become accustomed to it, then you can include a little jogging. For example, walk, jog and then walk again and it should be logged how far and for how long for each so that you can see your improvements along the way. We have provided you with some progressive programs to work from so that you can choose which one will be more suited to you personally.

Important: Even though it's great to have a workout partner, if you find yourself walking and having a nice conversation with your friend, then you can guarantee that you are probably not walking fast enough for the desired results.

How to choose the right location to exercise?

Outdoors
There are many advantages to walking outdoors compared to walking to a DVD or on a treadmill and the same principles apply for running too. Even though running places more stress on your joints, these stresses can be limited greatly if you progress gradually from walking to running over a period of time chosen by you. Choose to walk somewhere soothing, like around a lake, instead of near a busy road and do your best to maintain an easy walking technique. Boost the intensity of your workout by using hills or by walking on grass, sand or trails. To quicken your pace, bend your arms to 90 degrees and swing them across your body and take quicker steps rather than long strides.

Treadmill
If you're starting out on the treadmill, then 10 to 15 minutes is enough to begin with and the recommended amount is around three times a week. The advantage of the indoor treadmill is that you can also work up to performing upper body exercises holding weights throughout the period of time you are on the treadmill, and of course the advantage to using the incline button to work your leg muscles more.

In the home
If the gym scenario is not right for you and you don't really like the idea of people seeing you walking or running around your neighbourhood, there are certain alternatives. First of all, you could get someone to drop you off a set distance away and pick you up somewhere else. Remember, there is almost always a way around a particular problem or excuse. The choice of many people is to buy a fitness DVD. I remember a client who started to challenge her lifestyle in the New Year who showed me a DVD that she had bought and tried it out and enjoyed it. The workout lasted for approximately 20 minutes. The best part about her motivation and realistic way of thinking was that she already knew that this wouldn't quite be enough but she knew that the DVD also came in 40 and 60 minute versions. You can get out of these DVD workouts what you need and in time your body and mind will tell you when you need to do more. You will either be very bored with doing them or you will get to a point where your results have reached a plateau and you will no longer feel you are progressing. Our overall point

is… at least you are moving, and in some cases more than you were previously but you should continue to progress this over time with what exercise and/or activity you have chosen, until you reach your goal(s).

In the home workouts, you can use the DVD or a treadmill and you should try to implement resistance exercises, which we will explain in more detail later in this chapter. The underlying factor is convenience to you yourself, just as Douglas Brookes, author of *Your Personal Trainer* states "The opportunity to workout needs to be available at every turn in your daily schedule. It makes sense to be committed to exercise in a variety of ways that makes exercise easy, accessible and convenient. At every turn, the chance to agitate your body on a regular basis should be underfoot."
In the beginning, whether you are walking, jogging or running, you must keep your pace semi comfortable so that you can maintain it for a long period of time. We call this the active rest phase and you will understand this when I inform you of how low level interval training works. This method will give you a good platform and base to work from, as when it comes to working in short bouts (low level intervals), your body will be aerobically accustomed and will adjust accordingly.

Warning:
The majority of people on new programs start off too fast too soon and therefore can't physically or mentally continue, and eventually they give up. You must remember that everything you change in your lifestyle must be maintained and everything you do must be achievable and progressed accordingly. Giving up in our opinion is not an option!

How does interval training get you quicker results?

Any form of exercise helps but there are ways you can rapidly increase your body's power to burn food calories even when you're sleeping,. By alternating periods of intense exercise with slower periods, which is known as interval training, this exercise pattern fine tunes your metabolism. You can choose to walk, jog, cycle, swim or row it's up to you, and it basically consists of exercising for a set time i.e. one minute at almost your maximum capacity and then for another set time i.e. three minutes at a moderate capacity (active rest). You can increase the time at maximum capacity and lower the recovery time (moderate capacity or active rest). Within the next set of challenges we have developed workout programs that can be attempted when the time is right for you. If you attempt the programs and stick to them and progress them accordingly, then this could be the difference between losing weight long term or sticking to a diet that will keep you bouncing right back to where you started. The programs we have developed for you are only examples but ultimately, when it comes to setting priorities for yourself, if you choose three intense workouts each week, it will be better than five gentler ones. It's as simple as that and, in actual fact, the more intense workouts will actually take up less time (even though your warm up will need to be slightly longer to reduce the risk of injury). Don't toss the notion of long bouts of cardio out the window, but you should definitely consider adding short bursts of exercise into your day as a challenge. Maybe perform higher intensity intervals once a week. For example, choose a landmark, such as the end of the block, and walk at top speed until you reach it. Repeat this four to eight times on your walk.

Short versus long bouts

As with everything in the health and fitness world, there are arguments for and against anything and everything. But with the debate about short, high intensity workouts versus long ones, the debate has been highlighted by John M Jakicic and colleagues from the *University Of Pittsburgh School Of Medicine* in Pennsylvania, USA. Their results suggested that short bouts of exercise may enhance exercise adherence and weight loss and produce similar changes in cardio-respiratory fitness when compared to long bouts of exercise.

Note: INTENSITY is about getting the most out of your cardio in the least amount of time, so revamp your cardio program with new energising short burst intervals.

Why does building your strength ensure long term weight loss?

Did you know that you already possess the most powerful fat burner? It's your muscle. So why punish yourself and risk the loss of your fat burning potential? Adding just ten pounds of muscle to your body will burn off 62 pounds of fat over the next year, even while you are sleeping, and it will continue to do so day after day, week after week, month after month and year after year. Performing cardiovascular exercises at 50% of your maximum heart rate for a minimum of an hour was always the preferred option for a personal trainer to tell his clients and, in some cases, that is true. But what gets better and quicker results for weight loss?

In 2006, Stiegler, from sports medicine, suggested from his research that "strength training may have greater implications than initially proposed for decreasing body fat and sustaining fat free mass. Also, adding exercise programs to dietary restriction can promote more favourable changes in body composition than diet or physical activity on its own."

Strength training has the following benefits:

* Strength training builds muscle;

* Strength training turns your body into a more effective calorie burner;

* Strength training helps prevent osteoporosis;

* Muscle burns fat;

* Muscle is more metabolically active than fat.

Just to reiterate what you read earlier, if you don't want to go to the gym and you want to avoid intimidating situations by doing certain things at home, keep a set of weights in an accessible place at home for when you do your walking routine to a DVD or on your treadmill.

Resistant to resistance training

Toned simply means you have shed the fat that once covered your muscles and you can see your muscle definition which gives your body a lean, tight shape. The only reason some women feel like they look bulky is because they have excess body fat whilst building muscle and they are simply not eating in a way that supports fat loss.

You won't bulk up

Facts:

- If you are female, you won't end up looking like a man;

- Women simply do not have enough testosterone to get big and bulky;

- You will achieve a lean, toned and firm body if you do regular resistance exercises.

Realisation

Now you can start to realise what your body has to offer you. Your body is the answer to the results you require, why do you think yoga has been around for so many years? This is because it works. Try practicing some strength training yoga moves, such as maintaining the plank pose, which is similar to holding yourself up during a full body push up. The plank pose not only makes your arms stronger, but it also works your back, abs, and legs at the same time and it is something you could do absolutely anywhere. All of the recommended exercises that are within this book have an easier alternative way of performing the exercise and, of course, a harder version too. Lean, toned, fit bodies have low body fat and a lot of lean muscle because strength training maintains and increases your muscle mass and decreases your percentage of body fat.

Targeting certain areas

Most of us have someone we admire or look up to, but don't think for one moment that a celebrities toned arms or fabulous abs are created by some "magic" exercise that mysteriously melts fat off a particular area of the body or that they are any more happier with their bodies than anyone else. Now is the time to banish that myth once and for all.

1. There is simply no exercise that acts like a magic eraser to rid your body parts of unsightly fat, as that is not how the body works;

2. If you want to lose fat, you need to challenge all of the muscles in your body to boost your metabolism so that you lose fat all over.

Time saver

When it comes to fat loss, isolated, shaping exercises are generally a waste of your time and just because you feel the burn does not mean that you are burning the fat. One of the most effective ways in which to maximise your fat burning potential is through full body, short burst resistance training. By working several muscle groups at once, short burst resistance training has the following advantages:

- Saves time;

- Skyrockets your energy levels;

- Incinerates fat and calories.

Strength or aerobic training?

You should realise by now that you cannot achieve permanent weight loss with just dieting alone. Your choices are as follows:

- Diet plus strength training;

- Diet plus aerobic training;

- Diet, strength and aerobic training - advised for more rapid results.

The level of intensity during your workout will dictate which choice will work best for you and the method will have to be convenient to your daily life. You should now be in more agreement that exercise should be an extremely important part of your life and in some respects it is a must if you want rapid results.

The right mix

The specific challenges and progressive exercise programs that follow will ensure that your routine is well rounded, incorporating interval training (workouts of varying intensities) for at least three times weekly and performing a minimum of 20 minutes of strength training (using your own bodyweight) two or three days a week. The intensity level will ultimately depend on where you are at now and what you will be comfortable with. Being realistic is the key to choosing where you start, we can only give you the choices, but please remember one thing, if you push yourself too fast, too soon you will get despondent and you will more than likely give up, which is not an option!

What simple, easy-to-follow adaptations will get you rapid results?

Talk to your family doctor before you begin any type of exercise program.

PLAN A:
Your doctor can help you determine which exercise program is right for you:

- Walking outdoors;

- Walking on the treadmill and/or

- In your home to a walking keep fit DVD.

All of the above choices should be for a minimum of 20 minutes, at least three times a week or more. If your mind and body allows you to, you can incorporate some jogging with your walking routine for faster results, although this is your choice depending on your fitness level. If you choose to walk only, by the end of the 21 days (non-stop) you should be able to walk for 60 minutes non stop. Whether you choose to just walk or walk and jog, you should build up to incorporate different ratios. For example, "1 in 3" is equal to one minute faster walking or jogging and three minutes of active rest walking. Of course "1 in 3" can also mean 20 seconds of short burst work to 60 seconds of active rest walking or even two minutes to six minutes. We are sure you get the point. As your heart gets accustomed to what you are doing, challenge yourself further by changing the ratio yet again to "1 in 2" or "1 in 1," which basically limits your active rest time and you can ultimately keep increasing your short bursts as much as you can sustain them.

Important notes: Whenever you active rest walk, you must walk with purpose as if you are late for an appointment. We have termed it as active rest walking because it must be a speed that you can maintain for a long period of time. Never forget the warm up and cool down phases that involve stretching.

PLAN B:
Your doctor can help you determine which exercise program is right for you:

- In a gymnasium and/or

- In your home.

The most important aspects of these plans is good form i.e. engaging your abdominals throughout all movements as much as you can, also breathing correctly and maintaining good posture throughout the duration. It's better to perform good repetitions with strict body positions rather than rushing into something. Each time you try the exercises you will improve over a period of time, and practice does make perfect. Don't forget the warm up and cool down phases that involve stretching.

Resistance: As you are already aware, by working several muscle groups at once, short burst resistance training:

- Saves time;

- Skyrockets your energy levels;

- Incinerates fat and calories.

Below is a table that briefly outlines the exercises to follow.

Groups	Exercises	Time	Remarks
Ex 1a - c	Plank	Maximum hold in 2 minutes	Keep the back straight at all times
Ex 2a - c	Sit-Ups	Maximum in 2 minutes	Keep the knees bent at all times
Ex 3a - c	Leg Squat	Maximum in 2 minutes	Make sure the knees don't go over the toes
Ex 4a - c	Push-Ups	Maximum in 2 minutes	Ensure the hands are in line with shoulders
Ex 5a - c	Stair Step-Ups	Maximum in 2 minutes	Stand up with a straight leg every time

You should attempt to complete 2 minutes of work on each exercise, even if you have to stop and carry on. Exercise 1a will be easier than 1b and so on, and your aim should be to hold good form and maintain good posture.

Exercise 1: Plank pose progressions

Exercise 1a

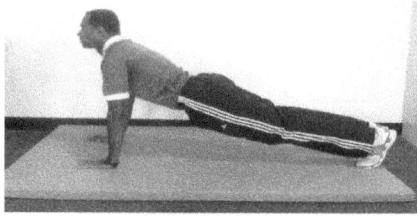

Hold your bodyweight up by your hands and feet.

Exercise 1b

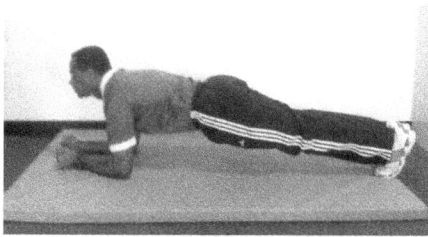

Hold your bodyweight by resting your forearms on the floor.

Exercise 1c

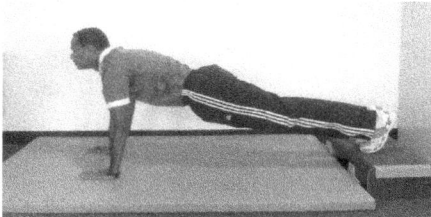

Elevate your feet on a platform to make it more difficult. Attempt this exercise on your forearms for more of a challenge.

Start - Start in an outstretched position as in all of the pictures.

- Your hands or elbows should be directly underneath your shoulders;

- Your feet should be together;

- Keep your back as flat as possible;

- Your head and neck should be in line with your spine and you should be looking at the ground slightly in front of you;

- Relax the tension from your shoulders.

Aim – To stay in this position as long as possible, just count those seconds and record your achievements in your workout diary!

Tips & techniques - Remember to breathe, pull your belly button into your spine for maximum body tension, and try not to let your hips drop or your buttocks to be raised too high.

Exercise 2: Sit-up progressions

All exercises start off by lying on your back with your knees bent and your feet flat on the floor.

Exercise 2a

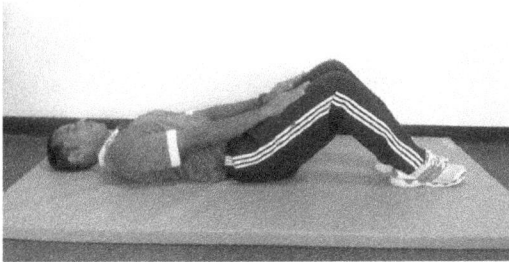

Exercise 2a

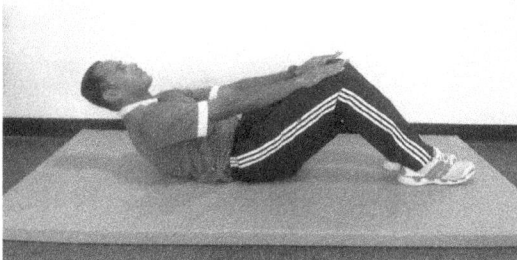

Exercise 2a - Touch the knees with the hands, hold for 2-3 seconds and return to the start.

Exercise 2b

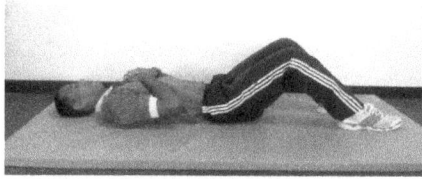

Exercise 2b

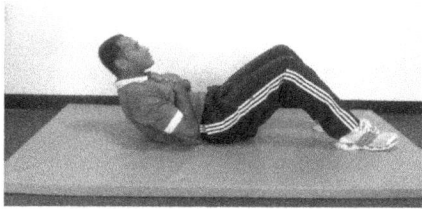

Exercise 2b – Keeping your elbows close in to the chest and your lower back on the floor, curl up so that only your shoulders and upper back come off the ground. Hold again for 2-3 seconds and return to the start.

Exercise 2c

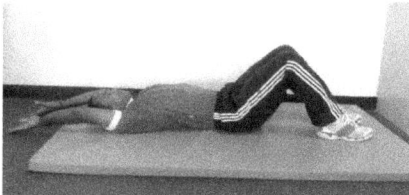

Exercise 2c

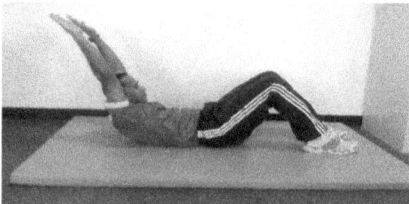

Exercise 2c - Extend your arms overhead, slowly raise your arms, head, shoulders, and upper back approx 30 degrees off the floor. Hold before slowly lowering. Keep your arms straight by your ears and in line with your head. Do not throw them forwards to help you. Add a weighted object in your hands in order to make it more difficult.

Note: To maximise ALL exercises, especially the abdominal ones, you can maximise the abdominal pressure by pulling in the stomach as if you are zipping up the fly on an extra tight pair of jeans. If you hold your stomach in whilst breathing out, keep sucking in the stomach more and more as you are breathing out.

You will feel your abdominals and lower back muscles contracting together and, in time, this will improve the support for your spine and lower back. This technique can be done anywhere, even while standing in a queue or sitting in your car. It should especially be utilised during exercise to accompany your body's postural alignment.

Exercise 3: Leg squat

Exercise 3a

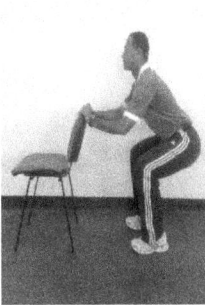

Exercise 3b

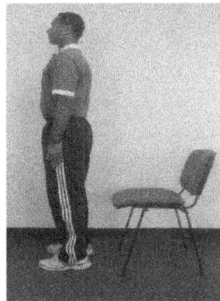

Exercise 3c

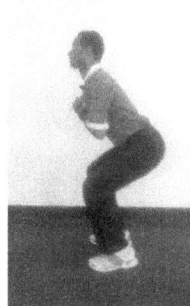

All of these exercises will tone the muscles in the back and front of your thighs and buttocks.

- You should stand with your feet approximately shoulder width apart, your arms either holding an object or fully extended in front of you for balance. Your toes slightly pointing outwards;

- Keep your back straight and squat down until the tops of your thighs are almost parallel to the floor at 90-degrees. Be sure to keep your weight firmly over your heels;

- Rise back to the standing position, making sure that most of your bodyweight is through your heels. The chair or alternative object should only be used as a guide.

Exercise 3c involves a heel raise at the end of the squat and can be performed without a chair as long as you squat down to a 90-degree angle.

Note: As with any exercise, you can progress it accordingly, especially the balance aspect, as it can be progressed by placing your arms across your chest and even closing your eyes, but remember to be safe. You can also add weights to your program by way of dumbbells or a barbell to improve your strength further.

Make sure that your knees stay level or behind the toes at all times

Exercise 4: Push-Up Progressions

Exercise 4a

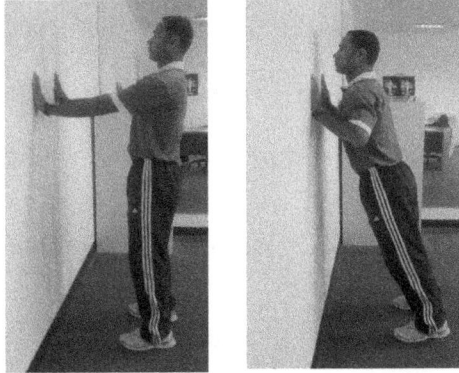

- Ensure the hands are in line with the shoulders and there is a straight line from your head, shoulders, hips and knees, tense the abdominals;

- Lower your body slowly towards the wall;

- Bend your arms and keep your palms in a fixed position;

- Your upper chest should be close to your hands;

- Straighten your arms as you push your body away from the wall;

- Relax the tension from your shoulders.

Try not to bend or arch your upper or lower back as you push up

Exercise 4b

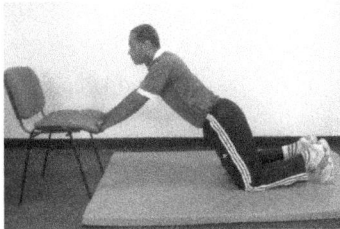

Utilise anything that is elevated off the floor, like a chair against a wall, your bed, your sofa or even your kitchen table, so long as it is secure. You will be testing your body strength more the closer it is to the ground.

- Ensure the hands are in line with the shoulders and there is a straight line from your head, shoulders, hips and knees;

- Keep the knees resting on the floor and keep your body straight;

- Lower your body slowly towards the elevated object;

- Relax the tension from your shoulders;

- Bend your arms and keep your palms in a fixed position;

- Then straighten your arms as you push your body up off the object.

Try not to bend or arch your upper or lower back as you push up

Exercise 4c

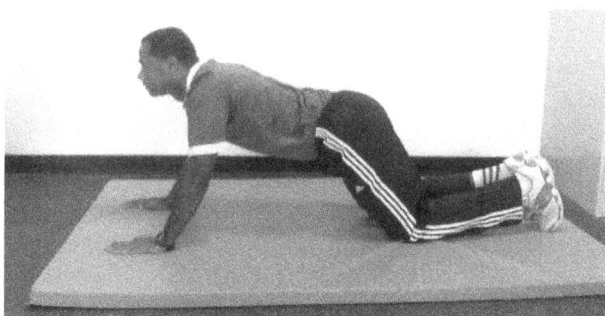

The push-up exercise has been gradually progressed against gravity and now you will be using the floor but still resting the knees. Try it without resting them if you can.

- Ensure the hands are in line with the shoulders and there is a straight line from your head, shoulders, hips and knees;

- Relax the tension from your shoulders;

- Keep the knees resting on the floor and keep your body straight;

- Lower your body slowly towards the floor;

- Bend your arms and keep your palms in a fixed position;

- Then straighten your arms as you push your body up off the floor.

Try not to bend or arch your upper or lower back as you push up

Exercise 5: Step-Ups

You can find stairs almost anywhere so make sure you do these exercises. In some ways step ups can be better for you than normal walking to get results quicker.

Exercise 5a

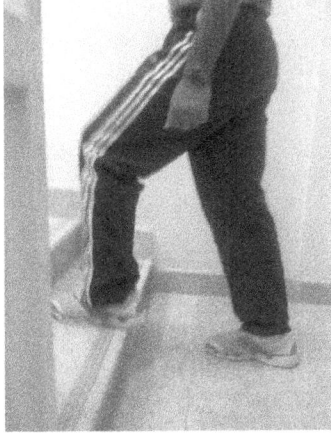

Exercise 5a is a simple step up and step down, changing the legs accordingly. Make sure you step up and straighten each leg fully, carry weights to make harder.

Exercise 5b

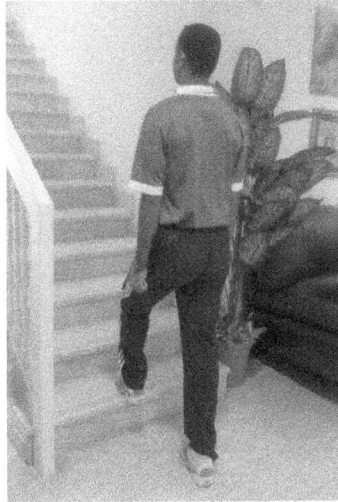

Exercise 5b is a simple walk up the stairs. Turn around at the top and return to the bottom, remembering to straighten the legs fully on each step. Carry weights to make this exercise harder

Exercise 5c

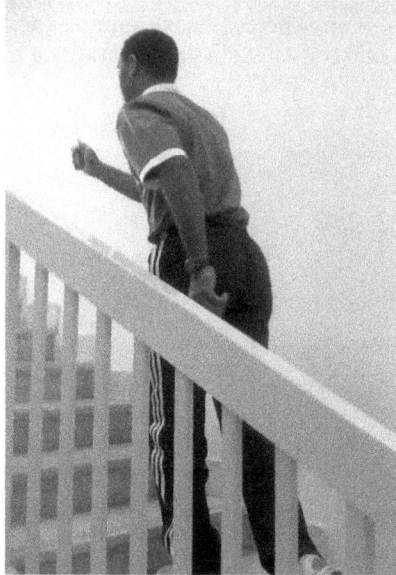

Exercise 5c is a simple jog up the stairs or you can alternate the jog with a walk up the stairs. Try and return to the bottom by walking backwards but remember to be extra safe. You are working your balance and muscles a lot more whilst walking backwards. Instead of walking backwards you can quite simply jog up and down for safety purposes. Carry weights to make this exercise more difficult.

Are you a complete Beginner?...if so try this!

Walking only program for 21 days (continuous) -

A daily/weekly walking log should always be kept for motivation and to ensure that you stick to your goals for the new you. Below is an example of a walking only workout program for 21 days that will get yourself focused on your new daily routine, whether it is outside or on a treadmill.

If you choose to walk to a DVD for 20 minutes, try and do it once a day at the start of the program, twice a day in the middle and then attempt three times a day nearer the end. This of course depends on the DVD and whether it includes resistance exercises or whether or not the time of the workout is longer than 20 minutes.

It's a good idea to get a bunch of DVD's that progress from 20 minutes to 40 minutes and then to an hour.

Day	Date	Distance	Time	Remarks on the walking only program
1	Jan 1	To local shops	**20 minutes**	Today I had to really focus on my posture
2	Jan 2			
3	Jan 3	On treadmill	**20 minutes**	Today I had to really focus on my technique
4	Jan 4			
5	Jan 5	DVD	**20 minutes**	My stretches are now becoming easier
6	Jan 6			
7	Jan 7	Around park	**30 minutes**	Started to walk with more determination today
8	Jan 8			
9	Jan 9	On treadmill	**30 minutes**	Felt good walking today
10	Jan 10			
11	Jan 11	Around park	**30 minutes**	My flexibility is improving
12	Jan 12			
13	Jan 13	20 mins out & back	**40 minutes**	Today I emphasised swinging my arms across my chest
14	Jan 14			
15	Jan 15	DVD	**40 minutes**	20 mins in the morning then in the evening

16	Jan 16			
17	Jan 17	25 mins out & back	**50 minutes**	My posture and technique has now been perfected
18	Jan 18			
19	Jan 19	On treadmill	**50 minutes**	I feel so much more supple
20	Jan 20			
21	Jan 21	30 mins out & back	**60 minutes**	Felt good for achieving my goal

I realise that it states a set time out and the same time back on days 13, 17 & 21. Although this is an example, you should endeavour to walk back at a faster pace because generally you would be warmer and more motivated on the return phase. Walking every other day will give you ample recovery time and you should look forward to the rest time. Ultimately, you will be more than ready for the next workout day. If your day dictates that you cannot workout on a particular day, you can walk on two consecutive days to make up for it.

Remember: This is a challenge for those of you who are complete beginners to exercise, and if this is where you are choosing to begin challenging your lifestyle, then you will be well on your way to changing your life for the better. Out with the old and in with the new.

Have you dabbled before?...if so try this!

Diet, aerobic & strength program for 21 days (continuous) –

A daily, weekly aerobic and strength log should always be kept to motivate yourself and ensure that you stick to your goals for the new you.

Overleaf is an example of a walking, jogging and strength program for 21 days, to get yourself focused on your new daily routine.

The aerobic work can be performed outside or on a treadmill but again, if you choose to walk to a DVD, try to increase the intensity accordingly to encompass the program.

Day	Date	Workout	Time	Remarks on aerobic & strength work combined
1	Jan 1	Walk	**30 minutes**	Felt good just walking today
2	Jan 2	Strength	**20 minutes**	Today I concentrated on technique for exercises 1a, 2a, 3a, 4a & 5a
3	Jan 3	**Rest**		
4	Jan 4	Walk	**45 minutes**	Today I walked very fast for 1min and 3 mins briskly
5	Jan 5	Strength	**20 minutes**	I can now do more repetitions of exercises 1a, 2a, 3a, 4a & 5a
6	Jan 6	**Rest**		
7	Jan 7	Walk	**40 minutes**	Today I walked very fast for 1min and 2 mins briskly
8	Jan 8	Strength	**20 minutes**	I concentrated on technique for exercises 1a, 2a, 3a, 4a & 5a
9	Jan 9	**Rest**		
10	Jan 10	Walk	**30 minutes**	Today I walked very fast for 1min and 1 min briskly
11	Jan 11	Strength	**20 minutes**	I can now do more repetitions of exercises 1a, 2a, 3a, 4a & 5a
12	Jan 12	**Rest**		
13	Jan 13	Walk & Jog	**45 minutes**	Today I jogged for 1min and walked 3 mins briskly
14	Jan 14	Strength	**20 minutes**	My posture/technique are now fine tuned for all exercises
15	Jan 15	**Rest**		
16	Jan 16	Walk & Jog	**40 minutes**	Today I jogged for 1min and walked 2 mins briskly
17	Jan 17	Strength	**20 minutes**	I feel so much more confident with strength training now
18	Jan 18	**Rest**		
19	Jan 19	Walk & Jog	**30 minutes**	Today I jogged for 1min and walked 1 min briskly
20	Jan 20	Strength	**20 minutes**	I can feel that my body is now one unit and I look fabulous
21	Jan 21	**Rest**		

Remember: This challenge is for you if you have tried exercise before or you just realise that the strength (fat burning) exercises will get you faster results, and if this is where you are choosing to begin challenging your lifestyle then you will be closer than before to changing your life for the better. Out with the negative thoughts and in with positive ones.

Are you accustomed To Diet, Aerobic & Strength Work Together?

A daily, weekly aerobic and strength log should always be kept to motivate and ensure that you stick to your goals for the new you. Overleaf is an example of a walking, jogging and strength program for 21 days to get yourself focused on your new daily routine.

The aerobic work should be performed outside or on a treadmill, and at this level you should'nt really be choosing to exercise to a DVD, but if you do, try to increase the intensity accordingly to encompass the program.

Day	Date	Workout	Time	Remarks on aerobic & strength work combined
1	Jan 1	Walk & Jog	30 minutes	Today I jogged for 1min and walked 2 min briskly
2	Jan 2	Strength	30 minutes	Concentrate on exercises1b+c, 2b+c, 3b+c, 4b+c, 5b+5c
3	Jan 3	Rest		
4	Jan 4	Walk & Strength	50 minutes	30 mins fast walk & all exercises 1b-5b
5	Jan 5	Jog	30 minutes	30 mins continuous fast jog (include ratios)
6	Jan 6	Strength	30 minutes	Posture/technique are now fine tuned for all exercises 1c-5c
7	Jan 7	Rest		
8	Jan 8	Walk & Strength	50 minutes	30 mins fast walk & all exercises 1b, 2b, 3b, 4b & 5b
9	Jan 9	Jog	40 minutes	40 mins continuous fast jog (include ratios)
10	Jan 10	Strength	30 minutes	Posture/technique are now fine tuned for all exercises 1c-5c
11	Jan 11	Walk	45 minutes	45 mins continuous fast walk (include ratios)
12	Jan 12	Rest		
13	Jan 13	Jog & Strength	50 minutes	30 mins continuous fast jog & all exercises 1b – 5b
14	Jan 14	Walk	60 minutes	45 mins continuous fast walk (include ratios)
15	Jan 15	Strength	30 minutes	My repetitions and sets are now high for all exercises 1c - 5c
16	Jan 16	Jog	30 minutes	30 mins continuous fast jog (include ratios)
17	Jan 17	Walk & Strength	60 minutes	30 mins fast walk & all exercises 1c – 5c
18	Jan 18	Jog	40 minutes	30 mins continuous fast jog (include ratios)
19	Jan 19	Rest		
20	Jan 20	Walk & Strength	60 minutes	30 minutes of each incorporating all exercises 1b – 5b
21	Jan 21	Jog & Strength	60 minutes	30 minutes of each incorporating all exercises 1c – 5c

If you think that walking is too easy for you and the rest periods are too often, then you can change them all around to fit in more jogging/running. But you should definitely try and rest in between strength sessions.

Try not to have two strength sessions on consecutive days. For example, there are two on days 20 & 21 but we have put that in because there is no strength for two days prior to that. As mentioned before, these are all examples of how you can implement walking, jogging and strength in a single program.

The allocated 20 minutes for strength can be increased and ultimately all timings can too. But this is why we have included the rest periods to make it more realistic as the rest time is very important so that your body can repair and grow accordingly and more importantly, so that your body can burn fat.

Your aim after this challenge should be to implement a good hour a day to your exercise time and if possible, complete a good five days a week with two rest days in between which will be dictated around your weekly plans. When it mentions to include ratios, this can be your choice i.e. you can choose 1 in 1, 1in 2, or 1 in 3 depending on how you feel on that particular day. The 20 minutes strength is pure work time and does not include the warm up, stretching or cool down but it's not bad to think that just by going through the exercise program twice you will be activating your fat burning muscles for only 20 minutes (actual work time).

Physiologically, you should complete the strength work prior to the aerobic work because large amounts of energy from the whole body can be expended while walking, jogging or running. Most of the bodyweight exercises are specific to local muscular endurance and will only use up energy from those specific target areas.

You should experiment and find out how you feel by performing aerobic first and then strength and vice-versa. It will ultimately depend on your intensity levels and how hard you work whilst walking, jogging or running and this will dictate how you feel when completing the strength work. Also, because some of the exercises we have chosen are specific to core strength, it is sometimes best to perform these at the end of a workout. Fine tune to your specific needs by how you feel. These observations should all be recorded in your diary, which you will need to keep, so that you can look back at your performance on how you felt.

Remember: This challenge is for you if you have tried exercise before or you just realise that the more difficult strength and fat burning exercises will get you faster results, and you will be closer than before to changing your life for the better. Out with the negative thoughts and in with positive ones.

How do you stick to an exercise program?

People are mostly under the impression that exercises help them in developing a good physical health. Few however, know that exercise can work wonders when it comes to mental health, especially related to mental depression. Sticking to an exercise program reduces the chance of various diseases such as cardiac arrests, strokes, cancers, and diabetes, besides lowering blood pressure and improving immunity and bone density. In 1990, a meta-analysis, which was based on eighty studies of exercise and depression, played an influential role in changing the general notion about exercise. When it comes to treating mental disorders exercise became the third most viable option, after psychotherapy and medication.

The research team, which included psychologist Penny McCullagh, PhD, made a few intriguing discoveries:

1. Exercise benefited mental health both immediately and in the long term;

2. Exercising is at its most effective at the start of an exercise program for people who are at their worse physically or mentally;

3. Old aged people benefited more than young ones in terms of decreasing depression through exercise programs;

4. Exercising affects both the sexes equally;

5. Walking and jogging are the two exercises most extensively researched, however both aerobic and anaerobic forms helped in treating depression, at least to some extent;

6. The more people exercised, the greater their chances of coming out of their depressive modes;

7. Exercising is at its best when combined with psychotherapy.

Weight can be lost in the long run by sticking to an exercise program whilst paying attention to the consumption of food in adequate quantity, and therefore burning off excess calories. All of these will help you to maintain a healthy bodyweight. However, you must realise that the ideal bodyweight varies from person to person and one has to be realistic by not always idolizing athletes and/or slim supermodels in their pursuit of losing weight. Workout schedules are developed only to help people achieve a minimum level of physical fitness, lower cholesterol levels and improve general health. Physicians must always be consulted before starting out on an exercise program, even more so when the person concerned is suffering from some kind of prior ailment.

When it comes to people aged more than 40, they at times need to go through a detoxification process if they have been inactive for a long time. This is done in order to ensure that toxins from food, air and water do not accumulate in their liver, colon and lymph. It is ideal to start exercise programs only after the detoxification procedure has been completed, less toxins get spread out all over the body while exercising. These toxins resettle in various tissues and cause damage in the long run. A balanced fitness regime begins with warming up and always pays attention to cardio respiratory fitness, muscle strength, endurance and flexibility. Stick to an exercise program and you are prone to losing weight in the way you want to.

Move forward with movement and avoid the health scares
Avoid sitting around and try to be the first one to leap up and help with whatever needs to be done. Sitting around not only leads to eating, but it also promotes an energy slump, which will lead to more sitting around. Try and fit in your usual trip to the gym or activities when you can, or go out for a quick walk every day, especially after a meal. Your activity or excuse to move could be anything to get the blood pumping and get you out of your chair.

A study of more than 13,000 men and women over an eight year period indicated that even modest amounts of exercise substantially reduces the risk of death from heart disease, cancer and other causes. Therefore, if we avoid movement, then the opposite effect will be produced and we cannot attempt to balance metabolic activity, which is extremely important with weight loss.

Main excuses about exercising
Only 1 in 4 people exercise regularly with the main reasons for not exercising being: Time, Boredom and Pain. Let's look at them individually but bare in mind that generally there is a solution to almost any given problem:

- **Time** – There are 24 hours in a day. You sleep, you can spend a lot of time working, but you can generally lounge around a lot too;

- **Boredom** - Prevent boredom by trying activities that you are interested in;

- **Pain** - You should only progress your exercise at a comfortable rate for you, and when your body feels that it has reached a plateau.

You must always be honest with yourself and if you have tried certain methods before, whether it be a diet or a certain exercise or activity, then maybe you have to stop saying "I've tried EVERYTHING" and admit that those things were more than likely the wrong things.

Light a fire
When it comes to metabolism, the value of exercise goes beyond the amount of calories you burn. Resistance training builds muscle and regular sustained movement supports your thyroid, lowers inflammation and improves the rate at which insulin can move blood sugar into your cells, so there's more available as fuel and less sugar circulating in the blood to be turned into fat.

114

Sweating
Toxins are accumulated through rapid weight loss, and when you burn fat the toxins it stores enter the bloodstream so the solution is turned to sweat. Your body excretes toxins and waste in perspiration and if you don't sweat, it can only be compared to not going to the bathroom. Regular exercise should make you sweat. Losing weight gradually without crash dieting, will also help prevent your bloodstream from becoming a toxic dump.

Prioritising
Prioritising exercise is essential for weight loss, but that doesn't mean you have to become a gym rat. You simply have to do what fits into your life, even things you can do at home, so long as you get your heart rate up. It is common knowledge to all personal trainers, life coaches and others that the biggest obstacle for anyone wanting to begin a new weight loss program is how to get started, whether it is too intimidating or they just don't know where to start. If you are already doing some form of exercise or activity and for some reason you feel that what you have chosen is becoming a chore rather than a pleasure, then you need to remember three important things:

1. Complete exercises and/or activities for long enough to feel the benefits;

2. Results will come if you work at them for long enough;

3. A calorie is a unit of heat, therefore you must increase the heat to burn the fat;

4. Try and find the right things for you.

Which time of day is best for you to exercise?

As we have already established, your body needs to move and this movement needs to become a habit, but it should be no different to any other action that has become a part of your life. People who exercise in the morning are 40% more consistent than those who exercise later in the day, and the key to long term weight loss is to commit to something and stick with it for the long haul and become consistent. When you're busy or stressed out, exercise is often the first thing to go, but you are more likely to stick to your plan if you treat it as a can't miss meeting. Try marking your workout on your calendar or set yourself a reminder. The time of day you workout depends on your routine but of course routines can be changed. Whether you get up earlier or eat later you can change, and that choice just like whether you want to lose weight successfully or not, will always be yours. Positive thinking and positive doing is how success is achieved and without paying attention to both, you may continue to struggle. There must be positive thinking and positive action.
It is important at this stage to remind you of the major advantages to any exercise and how it can significantly reduce the risks of:

• Stroke;

• Diabetes;

- Osteoporosis;

- High blood pressure;

- Stress and depression.

There are also several psychological benefits, including feeling better, sleeping better and an increased outlook on life in general. Many of the benefits and risks have been covered previously.

A calorie diet, with & without exercise...Revealed!
By now you should be realising how important exercise is, but to be honest we have only just scratched the surface. Where is the evidence to suggest the effects of alternating calorie diet with and without exercise in the treatment of obesity? James Hill and colleagues from the Department of Paediatrics at Vanderbilt University in Nashville completed a study using moderately obese women who were randomly assigned to an alternating or constant calorie diet with or without aerobic exercise.

- Both of the diets provided an average of 1200 calories per day over a 12 week period;

- The women who exercised walked five days a week;

- All subjects participated in an intensive outpatient behaviour modification program.

At the end of the study, exercised subjects had greater reductions in bodyweight and body fat percentage than the non-exercised subjects. Exercise was clearly beneficial in weight loss therapy. This study involved the behaviour modification program which would have included changing the mindset about junk foods, drinking soda and eating in moderation etc.

Important: It's not how many calories you can burn per exercise, but how many calories you burn 24-7.

Exercising is the best way to keep your weight in check, and a regular exercise plan is a must in order to be able to get in shape. By regular exercise we mean exercising at least 5 times a week. Strolling does not count as exercise, although brisk walking can be very effective. Eat at one specific place, most of the time we eat when we are reading or watching TV, so even when we are not hungry we eat as soon as we start to do that specific activity, this is entirely wrong and as such we should have a specific place in our house that should be designated to eating only, therefore as soon as you finish eating, leave that area.

After a short while of taking diet pills you will surely be wanting more food than you ever did before, you can also sustain serious heart and liver damage because of them. Also check on the medicine that you take and if you feel that it seems to be increasing

116

your appetite then consult your physician, he or she may be able to substitute it with something else. A weight loss program should be a lifetime change, you do not want to lose weight for a week and then again gain weight. In case of fad diets you should take extreme steps so that you lose weight but you cannot always go on with these extreme measures, thus it is important that you choose a diet program that you will be able to stick with for the rest of your life. If you really want to lose weight, a little bit of optimism and good habit change can do the trick, stick to one helping only, avoid fried food at all costs and say no to dessert and yes to fruits and of course regular exercise, then and only then will you be on your way to success!

A FEW FINAL THOUGHTS
BEFORE YOU BEGIN

"Failing to plan means planning to fail. What are your goals?"

- Brian Tracy

Be open to change

As human beings, most of us do not want to accept change and we try to avoid changes as much as possible. To cite an example, if the role of an individual at work changes, they might be hesitant to accept that initially, even though it might be a positive one. It has been proven that though people do better with changes, they are somehow not willing to accept it. The same holds true for our eating habits aswell. If you ask anyone to go on a diet, they will be able to do so because they are aware that dieting would only be temporary, and they would surely be able to revert back after a certain span of time. But if you ask them to undergo a change in their eating habits, they will be reluctant to do so. So in such cases, one can go for small changes on a regular basis for benefit in the long run.

Lifestyle change

The simple idea of making healthier choices with a single choice at a time for the remaining part of your life is termed lifestyle change. Avoiding certain groups of food and having a guilt trip while eating a cookie are pointless. Eating everything in moderation is the solution to managing a lifestyle change. Limit yourself to a few bites of irresistible food, or whenever possible, decide on healthy eating options. Daily physical activities should also be a part of a lifestyle change. Apart from being generally active through the course of the day, intentional exercises should be included too. Permanent loss need not be achieved by spending hours at the gym, as all you actually require is a 30 minute walk with some strength training some days a week.

Your lifestyle changes will make you feel superb and energetic while steadily losing weight forever without a diet again.

Positive lifestyle change

The presence of unwanted fat in your body is directly related to your lifestyle. The intense competition of today's world and the strain it creates on your system can be debilitating. We all know this, we are also aware that this situation calls for an immediate change in our lifestyles, but we are still reluctant to bring about those changes, due to time or the fear of having to adjust to something new but these changes have to be made to lose fat from your body. The greatest obstacle you have to overcome is your own mental blocks. It is a common tendency to limit one's capacity to change for a healthier lifestyle. Most people keep harping on the negative aspects, they are pessimistic about their possibilities to bring about change in their lifestyles and lack faith in themselves. To keep dwelling on the impossibility of the aims that you set for yourself. Many people think that they will never be slim because their parents were fat, this kind of negative outlook is plain absurd.

Not only is it pessimistic, it is also escapist in a way. This way the person manages to bypass the actual challenge or the ordeal or the fear of failure. The second obstacle is our surroundings and the people we interact with. Society imposes certain norms upon us, in terms of what we eat, how we dress etc. and if these impositions are accepted then one can never make headway, one can't ever change anything.

Fear is another factor that prevents change of any kind. Not just the fear of change itself, but also the fear of failing to bring about that change. Some people are afraid of letting go of a way of life they are accustomed to. They are also apprehensive about whether they will be able to successfully switch to a new pattern of life. This kind of fear is imbedded into a person right from childhood onwards and these deep rooted fears seriously damage their potential to bring about change
.

The following two steps are very crucial if you want to achieve the changes you aspire to. These are to ensure positive thinking and an enjoyable and fun life:

1.   Information acquisition
You have to be aware of the workings of your body, so information regarding physiology or nutrition is essential to make those needful changes. Only you will know the reasons for your past failures. This awareness will fill you with a new zest for living, and will enthuse you to bring about changes, endeavour to experiment with newer methods of losing weight. Read books and magazines and educate yourself about nutrition and weight loss procedures. Utilise informative websites like **www.wholebodyworkshop.com** or **www.weightlossdubai.com** which provide the latest information about weight loss. Awareness is important but it's not the only thing. All of us know the importance of dieting and exercise, but very few have the actual drive to do it. So therefore knowledge is not enough.

2.   Support system
A support system is essential for bringing about change, change for the better. A support system is indeed indispensable. Losing a huge amount of weight can cause an endless amount of stress and anxiety, this may result in psychological trauma and in order to avoid it you need adequate moral support. Those who refuse any help have to be very confident about their own will power and have boundless faith in their self control, but for others it is advisable to take the help of friends and near and dear ones. They might inspire you to strive harder and help to sustain your resolution. People around you, even though they might not be interested in losing weight might help to cheer you up in case of depression or low spirits. You might join clubs to lose weight, especially the whole body workshop community via the web board, because then you will be surrounded by people who want the same thing as you do, i.e. lose weight. Your probability of succeeding in losing weight will increase if your associates help and motivate each other.

Do your homework about weight loss programs

You can lose weight either on your own or under supervision of a trainer. Here are certain things that you should check if you are aspiring to join any kind of weight loss program.

- Does the program counsel you in changing eating and personal habits which have led to your weight gain?

- Does the staff of the weight loss centre consist of professionals like dieticians, nutritionists, nurses, doctors, exercise psychologists and other psychologists or therapists to keep your morale?

- Does the program give you solutions for times when you might get slack on your weight loss program and revert back to your old regime?

- Does your program teach you techniques with which you can make permanent changes in your eating scheme and exercise properly to stop putting on weight?

- Does your trainer adjust your food choices within your schedule or compel you to eat stuff you would rather never look at?

- Is your program flexible and does it accommodate the likes and dislikes and the wishes of the trainer aswell as of yourself?

- Is your lifestyle taken into consideration before setting your weight loss goals?

Some other important questions that are normally not asked about which you may not get too much information, but are good to know are:

1. How many people actually complete the program?

2. How much weight is lost on an average by every individual who has completed the program?

3. How many people have complained of side effects during or after the completion of the program? What have they complained about?

4. Do they take extra charges for additional things like dietary supplements?

Weight loss is basically nothing but a desire of the heart which drives you to achieve your purpose of losing weight. It is not a physical want but a mental one where you motivate yourself to reduce weight either to look good or for any other reason. Many people want to lose weight so that they do not look bad but hardly anyone wants to lose weight to look good. This negative attitude is not the right attitude to lose weight and will severely affect your body and your food habits. The most common of all is a visit to the doctor which has scared the wits out of the patient when he/she comes to know that if they don't lose weight then they will die of a heart attack. We do not say that with a negative motivation something will go wrong in your weight loss program but for a commitment that you have undertaken for a relatively long term it is better if you could motivate yourself in a more positive manner. But many time's things do go wrong. Have you noticed that the binge dieters never really manage to lose weight? It is simply because they focus on the wrong reasons and not on the positive aspects of weight loss.

Beat the barriers

It is not absolutely impossible to negotiate these barriers and change your lifestyle. You just have to examine your own lifestyle to fix upon the areas that need changing. The first step is to recall and make a list of the previous attempts made to change your lifestyle, such as exercising or changing your diet etc. then you have to think out the reasons why they failed, or why you think they failed. Maybe you could not resist the temptation of a dinner invitation, or maybe you could not devote enough time to your exercise regime. Second step is to go beyond the apparent causes and engage into an in depth analysis. Why could you not resist the temptation to dinner? Now think about the times when your attempts did not fail and compare why you succeeded then when you failed now? Such a method is called the self search technique and it involves a deeper investigation of one's own psyche. This may lead you to finding some very accurate clues as to why and how you can change your lifestyle. This technique is like a self-search approach to establish what may drive your enthusiasm for various goals. Self searching can yield valuable answers that you can use to set out on the path towards successful lifestyle change.

Discover realisation

Generally, health and fitness seekers think they can get twice the results in half the time. Some of the things they want are:

- Weight loss without dieting;

- Fitness without exercise;

- Perfect health while eating, drinking and smoking. whatever they want.

These above beliefs are quite simply unrealistic and will only set you up for failure. Weight loss is easy but needs a little of your effort. Perhaps the biggest realisation of all for most people, is that all the excuses in the world won't get them to lose weight.

Below and overleaf are some of the most common excuses:

a. I have big bones;

b. I have a slow metabolism;

c. I have a glandular problem;

d. My hormones are imbalanced;

e. I have a thyroid disorder;

f. My being obese is through genetic influences;

g. 'I hardly eat a thing' syndrome.

Often, the only difference between success and failure with weight loss is how much you want to succeed but, if you are motivated enough, you will have the strength to deal with any circumstances without excuses. You will find ways to deal with whatever life throws at you and, although you might slip up now and again, it hopefully won't be a regular occurrence. One way of increasing your motivation is to have strong enough reasons to succeed and make a note of the reasons why you want to lose weight. If you can find about ten good reasons why you hate being fat or reasons why you no longer want to be overweight, then you can focus on why you want to reach your target and visualise how good life will be when you have achieved your desires. Think about how you will look when that moment arises and of course, how you will feel. What you need to understand is that, for the majority of overweight people, if you consume more calories than you burn then your weight increases, yet if you burn more calories than you consume, guess what? It really is that simple!

Reasons for unsuccessful rate of the weight shedding schemes
We tend to escape from the actual facts regarding the diet medicines, the weight shedding schemes and thus shedding weight in itself. What we fail to understand is that acceptance of the true facts will ultimately lead to a practical method of losing weight. Here are a few of the infamous weight shedding facts and it has taken me 38 years to fish them out. Most of you need to be certain that no such diet medicine or diet measure exists that will assure you with absolute weight shedding prospect. It is only through your willpower and your desire that you can deal with and sort out the emotional troubles that lead to your obesity and thus lose your excess fat practically. Pay careful attention to the above statement as it is applicable to most of the people who are making an effort to shed weight. I have been studying personal development for more than 20 years and I have been a qualified consultant for 14 years. Hence I have realised that eternal slimness is achieved as a final development in all the people who wish to be healthily trim via proficient methods. Most proficient methods generally take years to show results. Almost all the treatment methods are not remedial or a healing process. Hence people who abide by these procedures will remain unsuccessful in their endeavour. It is essential for you to select your weight shedding measure as according to its proficiency. Inquire what the later effects will be. Listen carefully and also observe the counselling person in order to gauge their weight negotiation. Most weight shedding counsellors that I have met are themselves obese, and are above 50 years of age.

Sudden dieting fascinations result in failed weight shedding programs
As the reasons for obesity are very complicated, dealing with this issue is quite tough. The reasons that we are aware of are the emotional, psychological, physiological, the biochemical aswell as specific habits of eating. The foremost thing that comes to mind when someone wants to lose weight is to cut down on food and the more advanced measure used, the more charming the idea seems. However, this does not result in absolute shedding of weight. You tend to gain weight again since you have not removed the reasons for your weight gain. You need to inspect your agility first. In case your concept of work is to move from the sofa to the refrigerator and then back again to the sofa, then I am sorry to let you know that no dietary measure will be of any help to you, and you will have to exercise at some stage in order to get results. In case your metabolism rate is similar to that of an elephant then you will soon start looking like one. Training is essential to alter your metabolic rate, and an obvious fact is that a person will consistently become fat if he or she does not take up some physical training activity.

One reason for the obesity is the loneliness we feel nowadays. We tend to fill our stomach with food if we fail to fill our hearts with someone's love and affection. We also eat a lot in order to make up for the deficiency of sex or another human being. Food makes us feel fat when we lack these things in our lives, hence your extra fat deposits will not shed till you find love or sex or that human touch in your life. To alter your disposition and be thin you need to deal with these first because they are the root causes for your obesity. Several food sensitivities do not show, and most diet regimes do not function if a person is suffering from some food sensitivity and is not aware of it. The only method that can be applied here is to eliminate those specific food items from your meals. It is essential for you to identify the food that you are sensitive to or that food which causes some reaction in your body. Merely knowing these foods will lead to a decrease in weight, an aim that no dietary measure could achieve. One of the primary reasons for being abnormally fat is emotional disorders i.e. too much eating and literally gorging can be an effect of sorrow, solitude, annoyance, desperation, depression, disappointment, strain, unhappy interactions or personal relationships and also low confidence.

All of these factors can and will lead a person to binge and gain more weight. Admittedly food does make us happy for a while i.e. we binge to relieve ourselves of all grief and disappointments. The problem being is that this binging becomes an addiction and we do not look for any other proper methods to deal with our strain. So by actually identifying our reasons, then and only then can we apply better methods to conquer our emotional problems instead of eating immensely and growing fat.

Develop new habits for your Mind and Body

Recommendations

- Don't discount the role of liquids in your dietary audit because, if you are like the majority of people you may turn to caffeine to jumpstart a sluggish day. What millions don't understand is that it can do more harm than good as it boosts the production of adrenaline, another stress hormone;

- Dependant on where you are during the day i.e. in the house or at the office, it can get quite stuffy and it's easy to get dehydrated without noticing. If you always have a glass of water and sip it regularly you won't get the urge to be constantly making cups of tea and coffee, which will dehydrate you more and often lead to eating something alongside;

- Throw a cup of blueberries on your cereal every morning to get two servings right away or include two fruits or vegetables in every meal, like a salad with mandarin oranges, and then eat another as a snack. In this case, no matter what, you will get at least seven servings a day;

- With reference to vegetables, you can incorporate produce powder into yoghurt, soups and smoothies by adding a powdered vegetable supplement into your morning shake. All these added extras to make it easier are all available at health food stores around the world;

- Steaming vegetables makes them easier to digest and helps you absorb more nutrients, but just be careful not to overcook them. A good marker is that if the vegetables lose their vibrant colour, chances are they've also lost many of their vitamins;

- Your body has mechanisms for setting your weight where it wants it to be, which can best be described as similar to the way you set the temperature of your house with a thermostat. So the right tool for the job of losing weight is one that changes your body's set point, so you need to change your metabolism.

Other thoughts you can begin immediately:

1. I will attempt to cleanse my body of toxins prior to beginning this program;

2. I will eat a healthy breakfast to kick start my metabolism;

3. I will eat the right foods at the right time and limit my processed foods;

4. I will eat more than 3 healthy meals per day in order to lose weight;

5. I will carry a bottle of water everywhere, drink hot water and lemon or un sweetened iced teas for their anti-aging antioxidants;

6. I will eat lots of fresh whole fruits and vegetables or make smoothies;

7. I will eat smaller servings of high fat/high calorie foods or just simply replace them with healthier foods or eat them less often;

8. I will pay attention, enjoy my food and eat more slowly, not in front of TV;

9. I will not eat fried food or take away meals and I will choose my meals at home or at the restaurant more wisely by eating more grilled food etc;

10. I will definitely eat more protein (chicken, turkey and fish) on a daily basis;

11. I will remember that alcohol has many hidden calories;

12. I will make my snacks healthier with tuna, chicken salad, etc.

You should definitely agree to these:

- I will make time for exercising within my daily routine, and I will definitely get up and move around more during the day;

- I will walk anywhere I possibly can, avoiding using lifts or escalators;

- I can begin to walk slowly and gradually progress to walking faster and further;

- I can walk anywhere, whether it is at home on a treadmill or to a DVD, or even outside;

- When I walk faster I will walk with conviction as if I am late for an interview;

- In time my body will know when I am ready to alternate walking and jogging;

- When I have tried ratio training and I reduce my recovery time I can jog further;

- I now know my own body can burn fat so I need to do the exercises in this book;

- I will attempt the exercises because they are easy to do and then progress them in time;

- Even if exercising seems hard, it will become easier as I become more positive.

Do not continue until you have written these down or cut them out to keep safe.
You are now more than on your way to success. You are over half way there.

You should dispel the myths
Before we begin with this easy-to-follow system, we have to demolish, destroy and
quite literally get rid of all past thoughts about weight loss. Of course I'm referring to
all the myths, lies, unrealistic expectations and promises that you have been told or
have even heard about through others. Once these are gone from your mind and the
record has been set right, only then can you proceed further and replace those thoughts
with the honest truth alongside realistic strategies for your successful, long term weight
loss journey.

More myths revealed:

- Fad diets work for permanent weight loss;

- Skipping meals is a good way to lose weight;

- "I can lose weight while eating anything I want"

- Eating after 8 p.m. causes weight gain;

- Natural or herbal weight loss products are safe and effective;

- Nuts are fattening and you shouldn't eat them if you want to lose weight;

- Eating red meat is bad for your health and will make it harder to lose weight;

- Starches are fattening and should be limited when trying to lose weight;

- Low-fat or no fat means no calories.

There are many more myths out there but the most common ones were selected for you.

Once you have all Your Own personal myths out of your head you can then proceed to
release from within... your own personal reasons for wanting to lose weight.

The external pressure of adult weight loss camps
Some people need external restrictions and penalties in order to lose weight, and this is
why adult weight loss camps come in handy. These camps provide them with structure,
education and personal counselling. This way you know what the issues are and you
learn how to tackle them so that you can have a healthier and better life in the long run.
At the end of the day, you should remember that self confidence and an improved self-
image are a lot better than the actual weight that you lose because it can help you lead a
more enlightened life. However, it isn't really easy signing in to an adult weight loss
camp. For starters, it involves having to take many weeks off work, and it also entails
having to spend lots of money, but the hardest part however is leaving your family and

kids behind as you focus solely on losing weight. However, we would strongly recommend you to take it up if you can afford to, because it can be a rewarding experience. It can almost be like a retreat where you can focus on your health and diet, aswell as your outlook and lifestyle. It can be a great beginning to a healthier lifestyle.

Restraint may be key to adult weight loss
You can lose weight even if you choose to give adult weight loss camps a miss. Yoga and fitness classes work wonders nowadays and they try and make use of the link between your mind and your body. Your diet and your exercise regime should compliment each other and this can be very difficult to achieve. This disjunction between diet and exercise is one of the major reasons why both fail to make you lose weight. The trick is to keep at it, and not give up after a few half hearted attempts. Try to avoid dieting since it's difficult to sustain on a long term basis. How long can you live without the food you want to eat? There are weight loss camps which instruct how to lose weight without dieting. You have to focus and control yourself while on a weight loss program, and your motto should be restraint and self control. You cannot afford to indulge yourself however much you yearn for sugar or junk food or fried stuff. Learn to say no, although too much denial can create other problems so indulge yourself just that little bit, from time to time. A weight loss camp teaches you self denial and that is crucial to lose weight and stay that way. Also be patient as all good things take time to happen.

*Visit www.wholebodyworkshop.com to view how the plans are going for our very own project, a spiritual retreat which includes a weight loss section amongst other areas related to the mind, body & soul.

WHAT YOU MUST DO NOW

"The real act of discovery is not in finding new lands but in seeing with new eyes."

- Marcel Proust

Prepare yourself for success

Preparing to lose weight can be the most important part of the whole process. It not only lines you up for success but it also lets all those around you know that you mean business.

So, what can you do to prepare yourself?

- Firstly set aside 21 days (continuous and inclusive of weekends)

- Replace your kitchen with only foods that nourish your body without adding extra pounds, like fresh vegetables and high-calcium foods, such as genuinely low-fat yoghurt, genuinely low-fat cheese and omega-3 eggs;

- Purchase a case of mineral water and fresh limes or lemons to ensure hydration;

- Get rid of foods with extra calories, such as snacks like crisps, cookies and processed foods;

- Purchase some adequate sportswear, an exercise mat and maybe a set of different size rubber weights. Even a personal stereo to take you away from it all, anything that will make your start a permanent one.

Support yourself

During the time when you are undergoing a change in your eating habits, you need to provide full support to yourself. Even during days when things look bad, you must have a positive approach. Criticising yourself will only act as a deterrent in your goal. So try substituting the bad thoughts by the good ones. Consider this. If you told your best friend that are aren't exactly being able to follow the new eating habits that you have for yourself, how would they react? Surely, they would support you with words of encouragement to follow the path you had laid down for yourself. You need to tell those things to yourself during the bad times!

Distribute time FOR YOU

Before you shift your habits, it's a good idea to determine where your energy goes. You should draw your own pie chart that shows how you spend your time. How much of the pie goes to work, your computer, your family, your friends and not forgetting the all important YOU time? How might you reallocate your energy to make room for change?

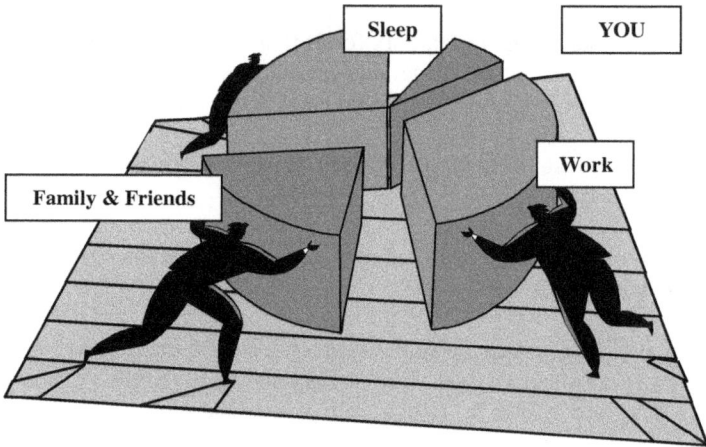

Make a little more time for yourself as and when you can. If it helps let people around you know what help you need from them, and how this will affect you when you are successful.

- The majority of people work an average of 8 hrs;

- We need to sleep for a minimum of 6-8 hours;

- Family and friends depend on your attention;

- Time for yourself is small, but ultimately you must have it.

Time should never be the issue for not being able to achieve what you want in your life. Remember, there are 24 hours in each day and that accounts for 1,440 minutes, so you can definitely slot yourself in there somewhere.

Release your reasons from within

Make a note of the reasons why you want to lose weight. Find about ten good reasons why you no longer want to be overweight. Then you can focus on why you want to reach your target and visualise how good life will be when you have achieved your desires, how you will look when that moment arises and, of course, how you will feel.

1.   I want to lose weight…………………………....

2.   I want to lose weight…………………………

3.   I want to lose weight…………………………

4.   I want to lose weight…………………………

5.   I want to lose weight…………………………

6.   I want to lose weight…………………………

7.   I want to lose weight…………………………

8.   I want to lose weight…………………………

9.   I want to lose weight…………………………

10.   I want to lose weight…………………………

Use words like "because I want," "in order to" and "so I can," but do not continue until you have written down all your reasons, or cut them out to keep safe. Trust me when I say that you are already on your way to success, you just have to have faith.

Example: "I want to lose weight so I can walk on the beach and feel comfortable without people staring at me."

Embrace positive thinking

If you have attempted weight loss before, only for the same body fat to return, or if you have had the same health problems with the same negative results, then you may have been unconsciously running old negative programs in your head and re-enforcing them with negative thought patterns.

Some examples of negative thoughts are:

- <u>I will never</u> be able to lose this weight;
- <u>I won't</u> be able to get into this exercise routine;
- <u>I can't</u> control my eating;
- It must be in my genes, so <u>I give up</u>.

Before you begin you have to demolish, destroy and quite literally get rid of all past negative thoughts about weight loss, including everything you have told yourself in your head or have heard from others. Once these have gone from your mind and the record has been set straight, only then can you proceed further to replace those negative thoughts with positive ones and a realistic strategy for your successful, long-term weight loss journey.

In order to successfully change your attitude towards food and drink you must write down a minimum of ten of your own phrases, phrases that you will need to repeat as often as you can throughout the day and throughout the initial twenty one days (non-stop). The results will be powerful, you'll see. Some examples of positive self talk phrases are:

- I promise myself to eat less fatty or sweet foods when I am tired or stressed;

- I will have more energy when I cut my fat and sugar intake and increase exercise;

- I will eat more high fibre and low fat foods that I like;

- I can eat often and still lose weight;

- I can handle stress without eating food, especially things I shouldn't be eating;

- I am willing to try a healthy eating and exercise plan to lose and keep off excess fat;

- I know how important water is, so I will drink more of it;

- I will become leaner, healthier and happier when I begin.

The prevalence of obesity has been on the increase and on the whole, improvements in patient education have not led to the desired outcome of weight maintenance, let alone weight loss. In more recent decades, behaviour modification approaches have incorporated strategies from cognitive therapy, which have involved the identification and modification of 'dysfunctional' thinking patterns and consequent negative mood states, hence the term "cognitive behaviour therapy" (CBT).

There is increasing interest in adopting CBT approaches to achieve more modest and sustainable weight loss and improved psychological well being (Liao KL, 2000.)

Your very own positive self talk phrases:

1.　　I...

2.　　I...

3.　　I...

4.　　I...

5.　　I...

6.　　I...

7.　　I...

8.　　I...

9.　　I...

10.　　I...

Use powerful words, such as "I can," "I will," and "I am," unless of course the sentence dictates otherwise. These phrases should go with you everywhere and try to place them wherever you can see them. These should be written down now or once you have read the relevant chapters, as this will help you immensely.

Example: "I will lose weight because I am more motivated now than ever before and I will not give up until I have."

Visualise how you want to be

When you hold and concentrate on a picture in your mind of how you would like something to be, it ultimately becomes your reality. To visualise losing weight you need to hold a picture in your mind of your ideal body, whether it is by using an old photograph or a magazine picture to help you visualise. The clearer your picture is, the more successful you will be and only then can you spend some time each day thinking of yourself as already having and owning what your image is portraying i.e. this new improved you. In time, this will bring you closer to your weight loss goals by working on your subconscious mind to achieve the desired results. Suddenly fast food, sweets, cans of coke and all those desserts will seem less tempting, and long walks will seem more fun, but only because of what is in line with the 'set point' you are visualising.

Basics of Visualisation

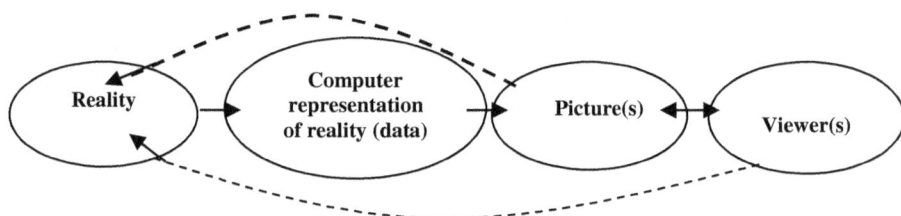

*It is critical that when you start these challenges and throughout the 21 days (continuously) and thereafter, you establish a new pattern in your brain by focusing on and repeating the following thought processes. Remember that your mind has accepted how you are today because of your vision, but your personal picture never had the opportunity to change until now.

Visualisation (Mental imagery)

Program the non conscious part of your mind and see yourself in your mind's eye i.e. not as you are now but how you would ideally like to be. If you do this on a daily basis and for a minimum of 21 days (continuously), this will become an automatic process. To make it easier, picture it as putting new grooves on a record by replacing the old (negative) grooves with a view that, in time, your old negative thoughts will be taken over by brand new positive ones. For ease, find pictures from magazines or books of what you would like to look like and place them somewhere you can see them on a daily basis.

If you have a computer, shrink or enlarge them and print them off and carry them everywhere with you. Place them wherever you can see them but remember, do not move on until you have done this. You will be well on your way to success once you have prepared your mind because your body will want to follow.

Set the right goals for yourself

The act of setting a worthy goal for something you have always wanted and reaching it through determination, discipline and hard work, changes the very fibre of your being and you become a stronger person, not just physically but also mentally and emotionally. Goals are very important with everything you desire in life, especially weight loss and if they are written down then this will be a bench mark for you to aim for. The most important part as mentioned previously, is the start date because nothing else can or should take place before this has been established. The only person that can set this date is you. You have to know that when you begin there can be no distractions from friends, family or anything around you for 21 days (continuously). There can be no reasons or openings for excuses, so choose the date wisely because you don't get what you want in life, you get what you deserve.

If you want success and achievement, if you want to lose weight, improve your health and transform your body, then set your goals and just go for it!

WEIGHT LOSS GOALS

Start Date: _____

My long-term weight loss goal is to lose _____by_____

My short-term weight loss goals are to lose:

1.   _____by_____ and
2.   _____by_____ and
3.   _____by_____

I plan to achieve my goals through these specific actions:
_____
_____
_____

The rewards for reaching my goals are:

1.   _____ and
2.   _____ and
3.   _____

Signature: _____

All of these new behaviours will move you mentally and physically towards whatever you have been thinking about and focusing on, so you need to make sure your thoughts are all related to where you want to be and how you want to feel and look. Your inner mind must change first and the rest will follow suit.

Let us recap on what you have achieved so far:

- You should have written 10 reasons why you want to lose weight;

- You should have written 10 positive self-talk phrases;

- You should visualise how you want to look and feel as if you already have success;

- You should have set realistic goals for your weight loss journey.

You can now set your goals immediately and make them realistic and suited to you personally. Your goals should embrace everything that creates permanent results i.e. the implementation of exercise and good food choices into your lifestyle.

SUMMARY

"You must be the change you wish to see in the world."

- Gandhi

Your past dreams are history

You must rise above everything that you thought to be correct before and eliminate all past beliefs from your mind before you can begin. You can certainly make gradual and small changes with your choices today in the here and now, which should only be positive. Your adaptation to today's society will help you become all that you deserve to be, but remember that any change is better than nothing and that all choices you make from now on are yours and yours alone.

Take just one little habit that you know is not doing you any good and change that one thing. It could be something like eating a cookie every time you have a coffee or piling the food too high on your plate or simply not eating breakfast. It could be forgetting to prepare a healthy lunch to take to work so that you have to go out for a Subway megasandwich or fast food. It could simply be eating beyond your point of being satisfied at dinner time.

Whatever it is you choose, just focus on one little thing for now and build on that by gradually changing your old habits for better ones. If you can, replace the majority of them over time, the sooner you can implement these strategies the quicker you will get the results you deserve. Do the best you can but remember its progress not perfection. Give yourself the whole 21 days (continuously) so that these thought processes and movement activities become a part of your daily, weekly, monthly and life long routine.

Remember 3 things:

1. Drastic weight loss means drastic life changes, which very rarely stick. That's why the weight piles back on afterwards. The 21-day challenge is the only way to begin to achieve what you desire;

2. Successful weight loss is in those little changes you make one step at a time, one after the other, until they become part of your life. Use these easy-to-follow challenges wisely;

3. You can start the 21day challenges at anytime, but you must be ready with no distractions and definitely no excuses. Remember that new year resolutions very rarely stick.

The truth of the matter is that no personal trainer, nutritionist, lifestyle consultant or mentor can possibly make any decisions for you now. The answer is already within you yourself.

Your new realisation and patience will get you there

A pound of fat is approx. 3,500 calories, so to lose one pound of fat in a week you have to eat 3,500 fewer calories in that week, which is only 500 fewer calories a day and not difficult at all. You can alternatively burn off an extra 3,500 calories and we have already established that this is more than possible with all of the challenges and their guidelines, by burning off calories by exercising or just by moving more.

Many experts believe you should not try to lose more than two pounds per week as this usually means that you are losing water weight and lean muscle mass instead of losing excess fat. If you do this, you will have less energy and you will most likely gain the weight back.

- **No brainer**
  The best way to lose weight and keep it off forever is to eat fewer calories and burn off calories with the exercises in this book. If you cut 250 calories from your diet each day and exercise enough to burn off 250 calories, that adds up to 500 fewer calories in one day. If you do this for seven days, you can lose one pound of fat in a week. It's easy math!

- **Influences**
  We are all responsible for how we influence others, especially our children, so by setting values, morals and lifestyle patterns, our children will pass on to others what they have learned in their environment. Such choices greatly affect our future health patterns and those of our children.

- **Justification**
  You must always justify your actions and everything that you eat, drink, do or think. Once that is instilled in your head (which it should be by now), then you are a winner. You are a success and you are well on your way to becoming all that you have ever wanted to be and dreamed of.

Burning fat and transforming your body is simple, but you have to work at it. If you're willing to put the work in, you will take out the rewards, but be patient because as you know all good things come to those who wait!

Combining it all as one

In this book we have been mainly focusing on weight loss itself, which is ultimately very important but what we tend to forget is that it is overall health that we should be focusing on. Even though contributing factors to death are all interlinked in some way, we should still look at the real causes of heart disease:

- Eating trans fats i.e. artificially hydrogenated oils;

- Cooking with heavily refined vegetable oils, such as soy, cottonseed, corn oil, etc. They are inflammatory inside the body and typically throw the omega-6/omega-3 balance out of whack;

- Eating too much refined sugar in the diet, including high fructose corn syrup;

- Eating too much refined carbohydrates, such as white bread and low fibre cereals;

- Smoking;

- Leading a stressful lifestyle;

- A lack of exercise;

- Other lifestyle factors.

Apart from smoking, heart disease and being overweight have the same contributing factors, so if this means making small improvements to your meals and your habits until they feel natural and a part of your new mode of thinking, then you'll surely reap the benefits forever.

When the time comes and your stomach is saying I need food, you have to give it something but it will be down to you what you give it. The secret to success for 'maintaining an optimum weight' is eating a little now when you first feel hungry, rather than a lot more later when you're truly starving.

Snacking is the best way to maintain your blood sugar and weight. Some people think snacking is cheating or ruining your appetite, but all you are doing is eating in a measured way all the time. Healthy snacking keeps you from bingeing on a huge dinner after starving yourself all day. Why do you think it is that you see the skinny girl in the corner nearly always eating? The choices you make, as important as they are, will reflect on how you feel and how you function. If you know in your heart of hearts that those choices were better than before, then and only then are you on your way to winning.

Enjoy moving -

- Instead of heading to the fridge, put on one of your favourite songs, grab your training shoes, and do a few sets of all over body exercises;

- Need a change of scenery? Embrace gardening. Mowing the lawn with a push mower and digging in the garden will all get your muscles working. Do anything you can;

- Maintaining a regular yoga practice can enhance your weight loss regime, primarily by toning muscles and reducing stress. If this is your new choice of activity, aim to practice for at least one hour, two times a week and varying the type of yoga you do, from gentle to more intense styles;

- At this stage you shouldn't be thinking of any excuses, you should be on the road to being positive with the smart strategies that you have just discovered, these are all strategies that you can start to adopt now;

- You should be thinking about boosting the intensity of your daily life with quality foods and safe exercises, complete with a good attitude and a realistic frame of mind;

- You should try and use your common sense at all times throughout the program. For example, walking up hills is better than on flat ground, and swinging your arms across your chest will be better than not. Swimming is an excellent method of exercising and great on the joints.

Why not try something fun whilst getting in great shape at the same time? Maybe you could start hiking mountains or take up cross country skiing, snowshoeing or downhill skiing. The activity you choose should be more than just fun, and when the weather warms up, perhaps you could try out water sports like kayaking or canoeing, or even take up mountain biking.....it's free!

Remember: Strength training has greater implications for decreasing body fat and sustaining fat free mass. Adding exercise programs to dietary restriction can promote more favourable changes in body composition than diet or physical activity on their own.

Here are some other weight loss tips that work:

1. Make sure you embark upon the project of weight loss for the right reasons, not merely to look good or impress others. Think about all the physical and psychological problems that drive you to over eating or laziness. Are you depressed? Or is it an eating problem?

2. Try and formulate a workout routine you actually like. Think about what you are eating, question yourself why you eat what you eat and when? then try and control it. This way your fitness plan will help you to retain your slimness;

3. Stress or strain at the office leads to weight gain, try and cut down on it;

4. You can impose the discipline of a weight loss camp on yourself, while at home. Check what you eat and stop when you have had enough, but control the hunger pangs;

5. Eat when you are really hungry not just because you are emotionally disturbed. Certain healthy habits can be cultivated slowly, like walking more or taking the stairs;

6. A support base of near and dear ones is a must to enable you to succeed in your venture. Colleagues or people who just like you want to lose weight, can make you stay focused and motivated;

7. A fitness plan is a must, but you have to chalk out your plan i.e. your agenda of how to stay fit in a manner that suits your body and your temperament. Whatever your plan is, stick to it.

Your mind and your body are interconnected, and it won't do to just discipline your body, your mind has to be rejuvenated too. Treat your body and soul as a single unit, and do not focus on individual body parts. The key to successful weight loss is to feel good about yourself and think positively at all times.

Your road to success

- Eat healthily regularly;

- Cut out the JUNK carbohydrates and fats;

- Eat good old fashioned home cooking and avoid take away or ready meals that began in a science lab;

- Baking, boiling, steaming and stir-frying are examples of heart healthy cooking;

- Stop eating before you become stuffed, full and uncomfortable;

- Never go hungry, you'll find yourself nibbling on everything that comes your way, so don't skip meals;

- Eat a piece of fruit on the way to the restaurant to control your appetite.

Remember that it's just the little things. As an example, the average person is gaining a minimum of 1 pound of weight each year, and did you know that this is the result of eating just ten extra calories a day? So instead of depriving yourself of all your favourites, continue to enjoy them every once in a while. It's the little things that will make a difference. If you must have butter, have it on one slice not two, if you must have your caffeine, get used to black, decaf or organic coffee. Stop at the tenth chip not the whole bag, at least it will be justified.

Calories in, calories out –
To lose weight you have to cut down on the number of calories you consume and start burning more calories each day. Calories are the amount of energy in the food you eat, and some foods have more calories than others, but foods high in fat and sugar are also typically high in calories. If you eat more calories than your body uses the extra calories will be stored as excess body fat.

Making the transition from a bad fat diet to a good fat diet is easier than you would think. All you have to do is minimise your consumption of meat, full fat dairy products, fast food, and products made with partially hydrogenated oils, vegetable shortening, and common vegetable oils. Keep it realistic and achievable at this stage so that it doesn't become a chore, but ultimately it becomes a natural part of your day.

Michael Van Straten, author of Super Energy Detox explains that "you should just focus on putting one foot in front of the other and you'll be surprised at how quickly you become absorbed in what you're doing, and that will be the beginning of the regeneration of your energy."

If you remember nothing else remember this, something that I will never forget my grandfather saying to me: "No one person who has already achieved what they want in

146

this life are any kind of superman or superwoman, and they are not special in any way shape or form. Of course they had motivation and the willpower to carry on, but we are all born with the same make-up." YOU have the same desire, just like our past clients, and now you have the same encouragement. Your soul aim should be to embrace everything that creates permanent results, with the implementation of exercise and good food choices into your new lifestyle.

We want you to be successful, in fact, we know you will be, but you yourself must believe, because if you believe in yourself then you will make it.

We wish you all that we wish for ourselves, and more!

FOR YOU TO KEEP SAFE

"To know the road ahead, ask those coming back"

- Chinese proverb

Healthy eating plans

Studies have revealed that if a healthy eating plan is followed, then high blood pressure amongst many other health benefits is reduced significantly.

Final tips for a healthy diet

Healthy eating is about feeling great and having more energy, not depriving yourself of the foods you love. Choosing the types of foods that improve your health, will undoubtedly assist you in reducing your risk for such illnesses as heart disease, cancer, and diabetes. Expand your range of healthy choices to include a wide variety of delicious foods, and have your own guidelines and tips for creating and maintaining a satisfying, healthy diet. Adding regular physical activity and exercise will make any healthy eating plan work even better.

Establishing new food habits is much easier if you focus on and take action on one food group or food fact at a time. Paying attention to what you eat and choosing foods that are both nourishing and enjoyable helps support an overall healthy diet. The best way to help lower your blood cholesterol level is to eat less saturated fat and cholesterol.

Control your weight long term by performing physical activity for at least 30 minutes each day, this is in order to use up at least as many calories as you take in.

Exercise works in conjunction with eating a variety of nutrient rich foods, and often includes eating a diet rich in vegetables and fruits, whole grain and high fiber foods. You should endeavour to eat fish at least twice a week and choose lean meats and poultry without skin. Cutting back on foods containing partially hydrogenated vegetable oils, and on beverages and foods with added sugars will all assist you in your quest to lose weight. Should you choose to drink alcohol, you should drink it in moderation or at least choose a lighter option i.e. light beers, diet mixers etc

On the following pages we have included some of the best menu choices for you, and these are examples that you can use during typical days, preferably alongside physical training.

Menu 1:

A menu of 2400 calories (for the days when you are not performing any physical training). Follow a similar diet to the one below for 6 days/week and then have one relaxed day. Look back to the chapter about Nutrition and follow the details about how it affects dieting and how you can achieve long term weight loss from eating certain food types.

Meals	Prot (g)	Carbs (g)	Fat (g)	Cals (g)	Fibre (g)
Breakfast					
1 cup fibre cereal (at least 5 - 6g /serving) 1 cup skimmed or raw milk, 5-6 sliced strawberries	14	64	1	300	7
2 whole eggs any style, 1 slice cheese	16	0	13	181	0
Water or unsweetened iced tea					
Mid morning meal					
¾ cup cottage cheese mixed with ¾ cup vanilla yoghurt, ¼ cup fibre cereal, ½ cup frozen berries and ¼ cup slivered almonds.	37	46	16	446	10
Water or unsweetened iced tea					
Early afternoon meal					
Whole wheat wrap with 1/5 Ib chicken breast, diced avocado, salsa, lettuce, little cheese.	30	30	12	330	6
1 piece fruit (apple, orange, pear etc)	1	23	0	84	4
Water or unsweetened iced tea					
Late afternoon meal					
2 tbsp peanut butter on 1 slice whole grain bread, topped with fresh berries	12	25	16	274	6
1 cup skimmed milk	8	12	0	80	0
Dinner					
¼ Ib lean organic meat (eye round steak, chicken breast, pork tenderloin, fish etc)	26	0	5	149	0
½ large sweet potato with little butter, cinnamon	2	29	5	160	3
Steamed vegetables (unlimited)	2	8	0	34	2
Mixed green salad with 1 tbsp extra virgin oil and 1 – 2 tbsp balsamic vinegar	1	10	14	164	2
Water					
Late night snack					
1/2 cup 1% cottage cheese with pineapple and ¼ cup coconut milk mixed in.	16	20	11	237	2
Totals for day	165	267	93	2439	42

Macronutrient Profile (Fibre excluded from calorie count)
Prot = Protein 27.1% / Carbs = Carbohydrates 38.6% / Fat 34.3%

Menu 2:
A menu of 2400 calories (when you are performing physical training). Follow a similar diet 6 days/week and then have one relaxed day

Meals	Prot (g)	Carbs (g)	Fat (g)	Cals (g)	Fibre (g)
Breakfast					
Egg sandwich (1 egg, 1 slice of medium sized chicken sausage, one slice cheese on whole grain bread)	24	30	14	330	4
1 kiwi	1	12	0	46	2
Water or unsweetened green tea					
Mid morning meal					
½ cup fat free ricotta cheese mixed with 1 cup vanilla yoghurt, ½ cup frozen fruit of choice (thawed) and ¼ cup chopped walnuts	30	48	20	474	6
Water					
Early afternoon meal					
Whole wheat sandwich (1/5 Ib lean meat: turkey breast, roast beef, lean ham, chicken breast or tuna, lettuce, spinach, slice cheese)	28	35	12	339	7
1 piece fruit (grapefruit, kiwi, mango etc.)	1	23	0	84	4
Water					
Late afternoon meal					
¼ cup chopped pecans, ¼ cup raisins, 1 hard boiled egg	12	32	24	377	5
Late Day Training Session					
Post training recovery meal					
Post workout recovery shake with 1 frozen banana, 2 tbsp pure maple syrup, 20g whey protein powder, 1 cup skimmed milk	30	67	0.5	386.5	2
Dinner					
¼ Ib organic lean meat (eye round steak, chicken breast, pork tenderloin, fish etc	26	0	5	149	
1 small- medium ear of corn	3	26	2	122	4
Steamed vegetables (unlimited)	2	8	0	34	2
Spinach salad with olive oil dressing	1	8	10	120	2
Water					
Totals for day	158	289	87.5	2461.5	38

Macronutrient profile (Fibre excluded from calorie count)
Prot = Protein 25.7%
Carbs = Carbohydrates 42.3%
Fat 32.0%

The first 2 menu examples are from Mike Geary, author of Truth about Abs.

Menu 3:
Sample Fat Burning Menu

Meals
Fat burning breakfast
Eat a small bowl of fat burning oatmeal, a couple of eggs prepared to your liking, a half a bagel or a slice of toast, a few strawberries or a few slices of melon. Add a cup of almonds, soy, or skimmed milk
Fat burning morning snack
Almonds and a small apple
Fat burning lunch
Salmon, brown rice, broccoli and carrots
Fat burning afternoon snack
A protein bar and ½ a grapefruit
Fat burning dinner
A piece of fish, chicken, or 1/2 cup of beans with a salad and minimum dressing on the side
Fat burning evening snack
1 cup of mixed nuts to include almonds, walnuts, and dark chocolate covered raisins. 1 cup of green and ginger tea with a natural sweetener If required
Drink water continuously throughout the day

Menu 4:

Meals
Healthy breakfast
Banana with 1-2 Tbsp peanut butter, OR 1 cup oatmeal with 1/2 cup fresh fruit, OR 2 egg whites scrambled with veggies and 1/2 Tbsp Parmesan cheese
Healthy morning snack
Yogurt OR 1/2 cup dried fruit and nuts
Healthy lunch
Salad with grilled chicken and avocado and 2 Tbsp dressing with flax seed or olive oil, OR a sandwich with Ezekial bread, lean turkey, 1 slice swiss cheese, veggies and honey mustard
Healthy afternoon snack
1/2 whole grain pita or 1 cup sliced veggies with hummus, OR 1 oz of cheese and a piece of fruit, OR a handful of almonds (approx. 12) or other nuts
Healthy dinner
5-6 oz steamed fish with lemon, capers and onion or baked chicken (sprinkle on spices and 1/2 Tbsp olive oil) with 1 cup sautéed or steamed veggies and 1/2 cup quinoa pilaf.
Drink water continuously throughout the day

.

Menu 5:
Sample 2,500 calorie per day (with exercise)

Meals
Healthy breakfast
1 cup bran flakes, 1 cup 1% milk, 1 medium peach, 1 whole wheat toast and 1 tbsp peanut butter
Healthy morning snack
1 cup strawberries, 1 small cup low fat yogurt, 1 small scoop (2oz) vanilla protein powder, 1 cup 1% milk and 1 small cup of orange juice
Healthy lunch
Peach Chicken and Rice, 2 oz skinless chicken breast, small can sliced peaches, small tsp of cornstarch, small tsp peeled and grated ginger, 1/4 tsp salt, 1/4 cup water chestnuts, small cup rice (uncooked). Small cup of snow peas and a small tsp extra virgin olive oil
Healthy afternoon snack
3/4 cup 1% cottage cheese, small can (4oz) of can peaches- sliced, 1small muffin and 1 small tbsp of peanut butter
Healthy dinner
Chicken meal - 4 oz skinless chicken breasts, 1/3 cup of low fat sauce, 1/3 cup orange juice, 1 tsp cornstarch, 1/3 tsp ginger, a small tbsp of extra virgin olive oil, 1 cup of broccoli florets, 1 can (8 ounces) of sliced water chestnuts 1/4 cup rice (cooked)
Drink water continuously throughout the day

Your post workout meal
Power Drink - 1 scoop protein powder (2oz), 1 cup orange juice, 1 medium banana, 1 cup 1% milk and a small tbsp of honey.

Menu 6:
Sample 3,500 calorie per day (with exercise)

Meals
Healthy breakfast
1 sliced peach, 1 cup low fat vanilla yogurt, 1 scoop (2 oz) vanilla protein powder, small cup of blueberries, small whole wheat bagel and 1 small tbsp light cream cheese
Healthy morning snack
1 cup strawberries, 1 cup low fat yogurt, 1 scoop (2oz) vanilla protein powder, 1 cup 1% milk and 1 cup orange juice
Healthy lunch
Tuna Sandwich, small tin of tuna, 2 whole wheat slices of bread, 1/4 cup diced celery, 2 tbsp light mayonnaise, 1/4 cup brown rice, 1 tsp light mayonnaise, 2 romaine lettuce leaves, 1 cup cucumber, 1 tbsp chopped parsley, 1 tbsp chopped chives and 1 cube of soup base
Healthy dinner
1 whole wheat bagel, 1 tbsp peanut butter, 1 cup cottage cheese and a small cup of strawberries
Healthy dinner
Chicken Teriyaki, 4 oz skinless chicken breasts, 1/3 cup low sodium teriyaki sauce, 1/3 cup orange juice, 1 tsp cornstarch, 1/3 tsp ginger, small tbsp of extra virgin olive oil, 1 cup of broccoli florets, 1 can (8oz) sliced water chestnuts and a small cup of rice (cooked)
Drink water continuously throughout the day

Post workout meal
Power Drink - 1 scoop of protein powder (2oz), 1 cup of orange juice, 1 medium banana, 1 cup of 1% milk and a tbsp of honey.

Low-calorie fat loss drinks (snack/lunch alternatives)

These drink choices are all high in protein and fibre, yet low in fat.

Strawberry Protein Smoothie
1 cup frozen strawberries
1/2 cup organic plain low-fat yogurt
1/2 – 1 cup of cold water
1 scoop whey protein isolate
1 tbsp of spectrum organic flaxseed (ground)
1 packet of stevia (optional)
Net Calories: 315

Mango or Blueberry Protein Smoothie
1 cup frozen mango cubes or 1 cup of frozen blueberries
1/2 cup of organic plain low-fat yogurt
1/2 – 1 cup of cold water
1 scoop of whey protein isolate
1 tbsp of spectrum organic flaxseed (ground)
1 packet of stevia (optional)
Net Calories: 355

Peach Protein Smoothie
1 cup of frozen peach slices
1/2 cup of organic plain low-fat yogurt
1/2 – 1 cup of cold water
1 scoop of whey protein isolate
1 tbsp of spectrum organic Flaxseed (ground)
1 packet of stevia (optional)
Net Calories: 315

Choco-Almond Butter Protein Smoothie
1/2 medium banana
1 cup of cold water
1/2 cup of organic frozen yogurt, non-fat, chocolate
1 scoop of whey chocolate protein
1 tbsp organic almond butter
2-4 ice cubes
1 packet of stevia (optional)
Net Calories: 370

EXERCISE LIBRARY

Using your bodyweight only

All of these exercises, workout programs and more up-to-date specialist content can be found in our other books **"Exercise Your Whole Body at Home" & "Maximise Your Fitness Potential"...** Just visit www.amazon.com or visit:

info@wholebodyworkshop.com
www.wholebodyworkshop.com

Exercise 1.1 – Seated back extension

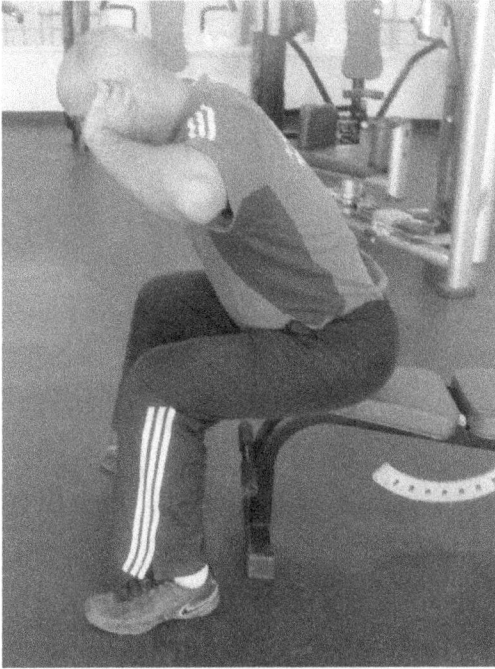

EXERCISE DESCRIPTION

From the seated position ensure that your feet are flat on the floor and that your hips, shoulders, head and eyes are inline. Lean forwards under the control of your abdominals whilst breathing in, under control move your upper body backwards contracting the lower back muscles whilst breathing out. Repeat the movement in a controlled manner.

Exercise 1.2 – Standing back extension

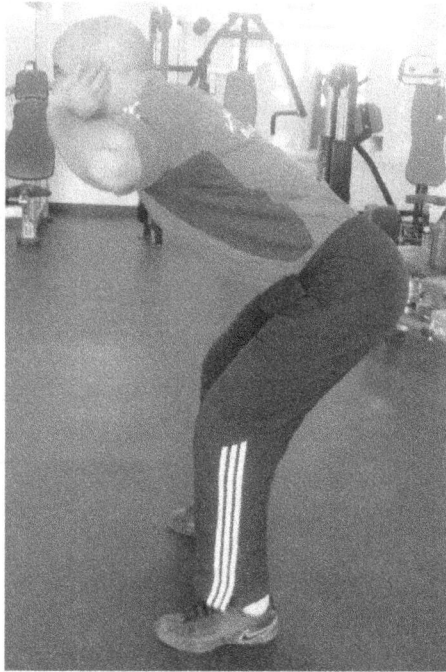

EXERCISE DESCRIPTION

From the standing position ensure that your feet are shoulder width apart and flat on the floor and that your hips, shoulders, head and eyes are inline. Lean forwards under the control of your abdominals whilst breathing in, under control move your upper body backwards contracting the lower back muscles whilst breathing out. Repeat the movement in a controlled manner.

Exercise 1.3 – Alternate arm & leg raise 1

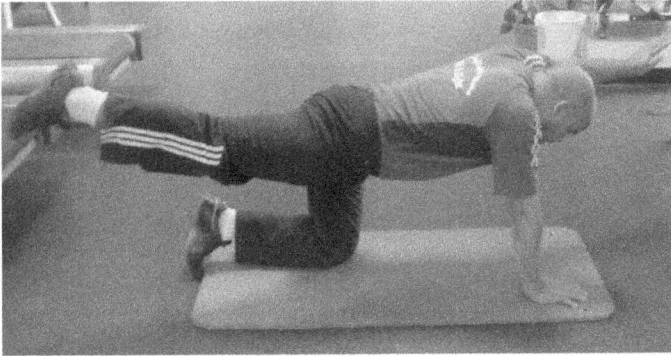

EXERCISE DESCRIPTION

From the kneeling position ensure that your hands are level with your shoulders and your knees and hands are in line. Your shoulders should be relaxed and your hips and shoulders should remain facing towards the ground along with your head and eyes. Initiate the movement from the abdominals and raise one arm and the opposite leg simultaneously whilst looking forwards as you breathe out. Hold the position as if you are balancing something on your back and slowly return to the start position whilst breathing in. Repeat the movement with the opposite arm and leg in a controlled manner. If this is too difficult you can begin by moving one arm or one leg only and then progress accordingly. Maintaining control throughout the movement is key whilst breathing correctly.

Exercise 1.4 – Alternate arm & leg raise 2

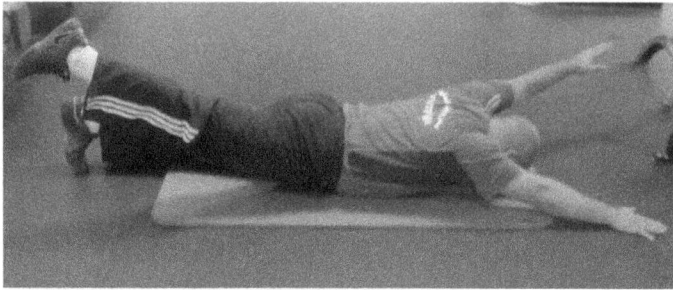

EXERCISE DESCRIPTION

From the lying position ensure that your shoulders are relaxed and your hips and shoulders remain facing towards the ground along with your head and eyes. Initiate the movement from the abdominals and raise one arm and the opposite leg simultaneously whilst looking forwards as you breathe out. Hold the position as if you are balancing something on your back and slowly return to the start position whilst breathing in. Repeat the movement with the opposite arm and leg in a controlled manner. If this is too difficult you can begin by moving one arm or one leg only, then both arms only and then both legs only. You can then progress accordingly as explained above. Maintaining control throughout the movement is the key whilst breathing correctly.

Exercise 1.5 – Straight leg hold

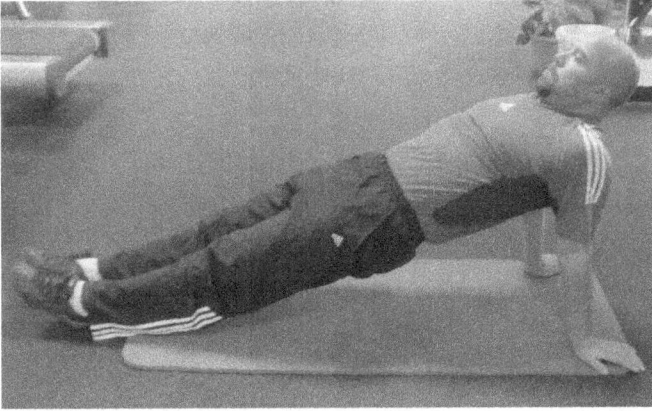

EXERCISE DESCRIPTION

Start off by sitting on the floor with your legs outstretched, place your hands level with your shoulders and ensure and that your hips, shoulders, head and eyes are inline. Ensuring that your hands are flat on the floor, support your bodyweight as you raise your hips off the ground whilst breathing out. Hold the position as you contract both your abdominals and lower back, return to the start position under control whilst breathing in. Repeat the movement accordingly

Exercise 1.6 – Plank progressions

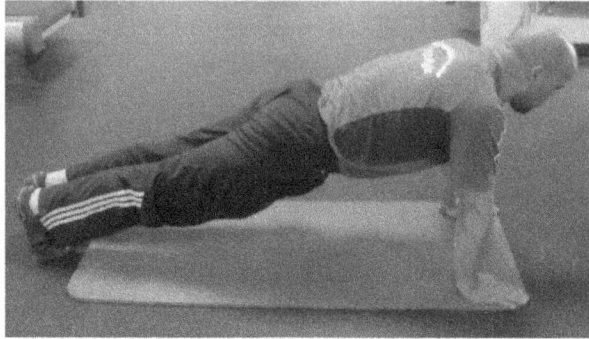

EXERCISE DESCRIPTION

From the kneeling position ensure that your hands are level with your shoulders and your knees and hands are in line. Your shoulders should be relaxed and your hips and shoulders should remain facing towards the ground along with your head and eyes. Initiate the movement from the abdominals and move your legs to the rear whilst looking forwards as you breathe out. Hold the position as if you are balancing something on your back and breathe in and out in a controlled manner. Hold the position for as long as possible but you should aim to work towards 2 minutes. As you tire concentrate on your breathing whilst compressing your abdominals and lower back, tense your whole body (not shoulders) to assist you in keeping good form. If you need to rest, slowly return to the start position and repeat the movement in a controlled manner. If this is too difficult you can begin by placing your hands on a raised (secure) platform and do the same as above. You can make it more difficult by doing the same movement but on your forearms ensuring your elbows are level with your shoulders and also progress by placing your legs on a raised (secure) platform. Maintaining control throughout the movement is important whilst breathing correctly.

Exercise 1.7 – Hip raises

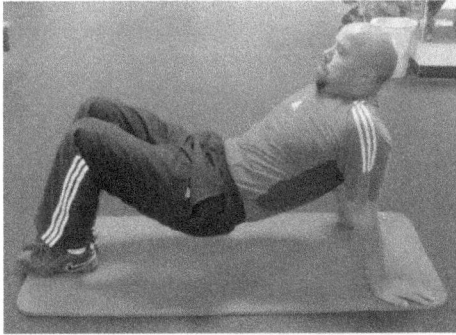

EXERCISE DESCRIPTION

Start off by sitting on the floor with your knees bent and feet flat on the floor, place your hands level with your shoulders and ensure your hips and shoulders are facing forwards along with your head and eyes. Ensuring that your hands are flat on the floor, support your bodyweight as you raise your hips off the ground whilst breathing out. Hold the position as you contract your abdominals lower back and Glutes. Return to the start position under control whilst breathing in, repeat the movement accordingly.

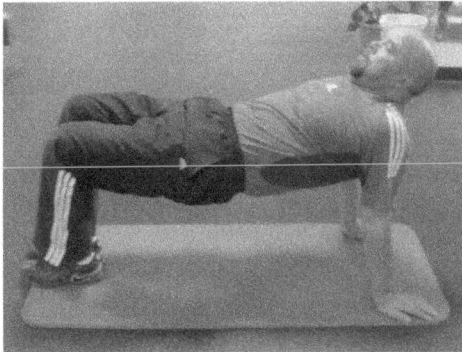

Chest

Exercise 2.1 – Pectoral Isometric hold

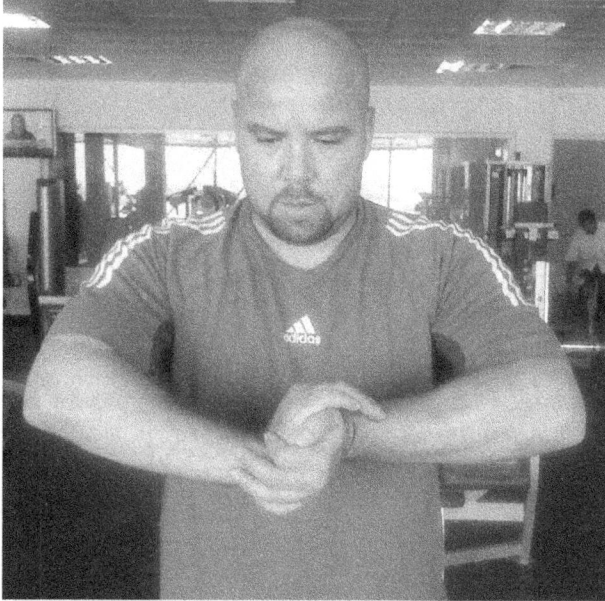

EXERCISE DESCRIPTION

Place your hands together & level with your chest and ensure that your shoulders are relaxed whilst pushing your hands towards each other. Breathe consistently whilst pushing harder and contract your abdominals accordingly to ensure that you increase the power for better results. Your hands should only be slightly in front of your body.

Exercise 2.2 – Incline Push Ups

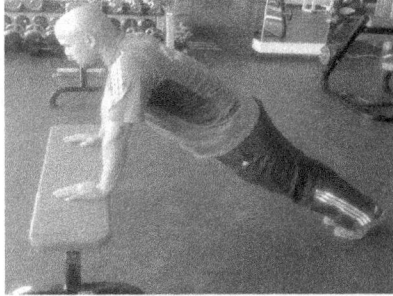

EXERCISE DESCRIPTION

Lean onto a bench/stable object ensuring that your back is straight and your hands are level with your shoulders. Your shoulders should be relaxed and your hips and shoulders should remain facing towards the ground along with your head and eyes. Initiate the movement from the abdominals and lower your upper body until your chest is close to the bench/stable object whilst breathing in. Breathe out as you raise your upper body back to the start position. Maintaining control throughout the movement is important whilst breathing correctly.

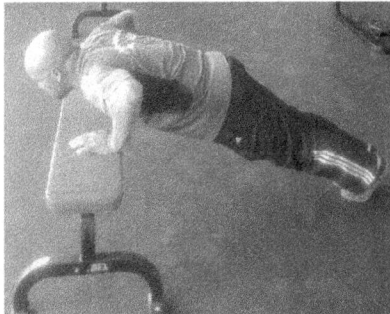

Exercise 2.3 – Normal Push Ups

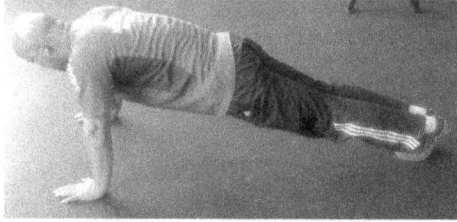

EXERCISE DESCRIPTION

From the kneeling position ensure that your hands are level with your shoulders and your knees and hands are in line. Your shoulders should be relaxed and your hips and shoulders should remain facing towards the ground along with your head and eyes. Initiate the movement from the abdominals and lower your upper body until your chest is close to the floor whilst breathing in. Breathe out as you raise your upper body back to the start position.

As you tire, concentrate on your breathing whilst compressing your abdominals and lower back; tense your whole body (not shoulders) to assist you in keeping good form. If this is too easy you can raise up from the floor whilst attempting to clap your hands together and return safely to the start position. Maintaining control throughout the movement is important whilst breathing correctly.

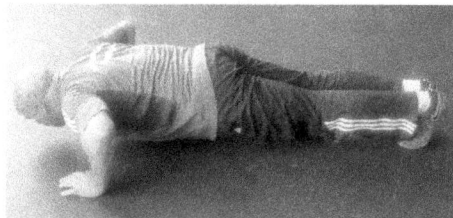

Exercise 2.4 – Decline Push Ups

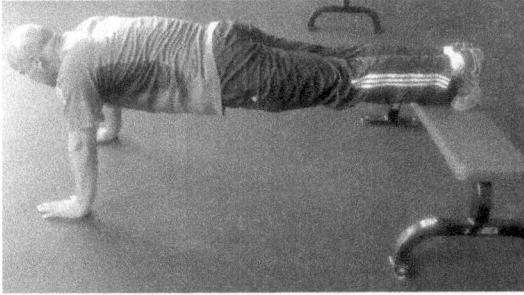

EXERCISE DESCRIPTION

With your feet on a stable raised object ensure your hands are level with your shoulders and your knees and hands are in line. Your shoulders should be relaxed and your hips and shoulders should remain facing towards the ground along with your head and eyes. Initiate the movement from the abdominals and lower your upper body until your chest is close to the floor whilst breathing in. Breathe out as you raise your upper body back to the start position. Maintaining control throughout the movement is important whilst breathing correctly.

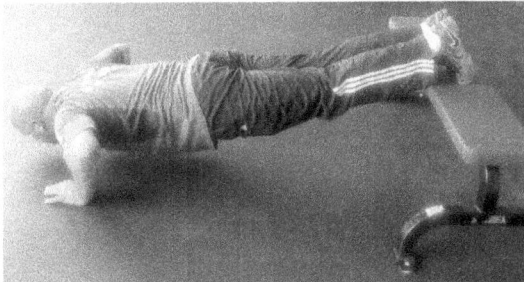

Exercise 2.5 – Bodyweight Dips

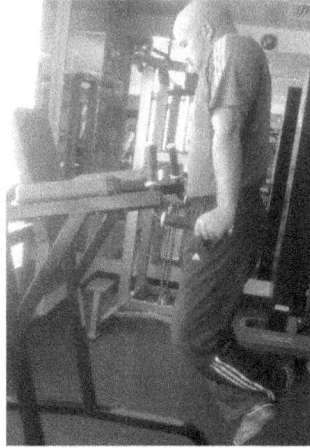

EXERCISE DESCRIPTION

Find any object that is stable, safe and secure where you can bend your elbows fully behind your body. Your aim is to place the chest in a fully stretched position before raising your body upwards whilst breathing out and straightening your arms. You can use the apparatus above or place a chair/raised platform behind you and complete the same exercise, although the above apparatus is better to get primary results for the chest as opposed to chest and triceps.

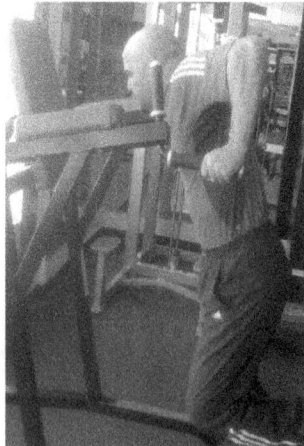

Shoulders

Exercise 3.1 – Isometric Holds 1-4

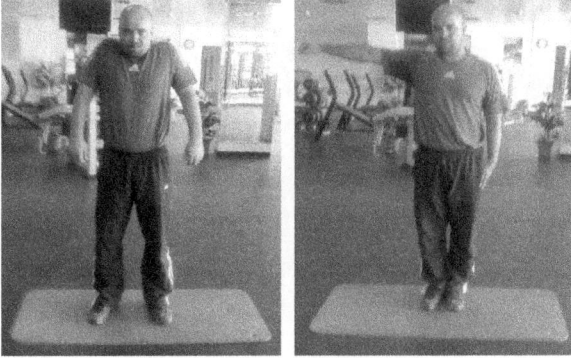

EXERCISE DESCRIPTION

Whichever hold you are doing you must ensure that wherever possible your posture is good i.e. maintaining body alignment with your head, eyes, shoulders and hips inline and facing forwards as much as possible. Your abdominals should be initiated prior and during each hold with your shoulders relaxed as much as possible. All of the above movements are shoulder muscle actions; therefore all you are doing is moving the arm(s) in a particular direction and placing a hold within the range, your breathing should remain controlled and should not be forced.

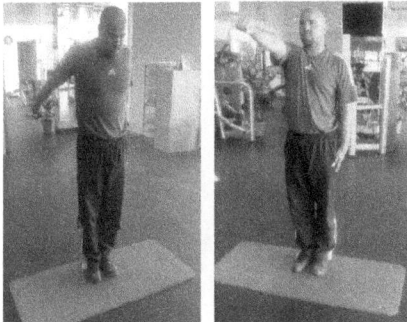

Exercise 3.2 – Advanced Hold

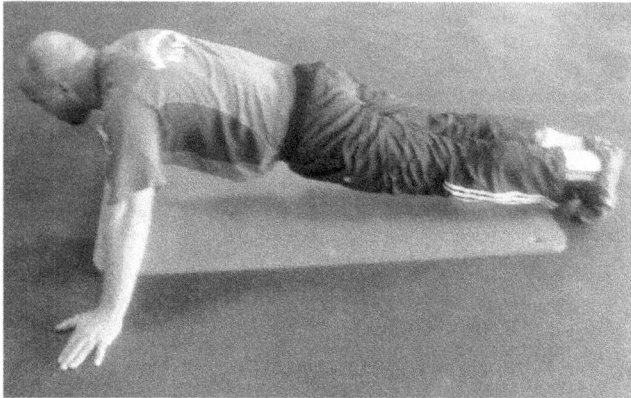

EXERCISE DESCRIPTION

With this hold you must ensure that your posture is perfect i.e. maintaining body alignment with your head, eyes, shoulders and hips inline and facing forwards as much as possible. Your abdominals should be initiated prior and during the hold with your shoulders relaxed as much as possible. Your hands should be inline with the shoulders and your breathing should remain controlled and should not be forced. Hold the position for as long as possible without disrupting your body alignment and good form.

Exercise 3.3 – Partner Resisted Exercises

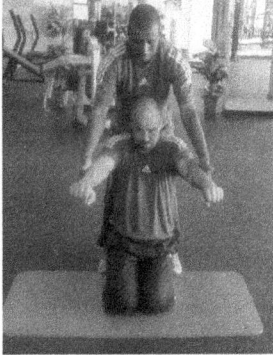 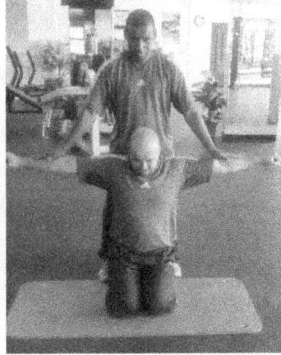

Pull arms down   Push arms up

EXERCISE DESCRIPTION

Most of the exercises shown are a variation of all the movements already covered (3.1), whether you are standing, or kneeling, your partner is just applying a resistance within a certain range whilst you attempt to raise, lower, push or pull against that resistance. You should always continue to breathe naturally and maintain good posture and form.

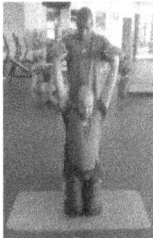 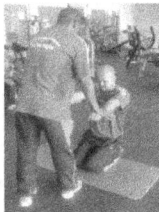 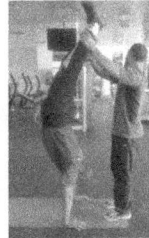

Push arms up   Push arms up   Hold or
                                Bend & Push

Exercise 3.4 – Caterpillar

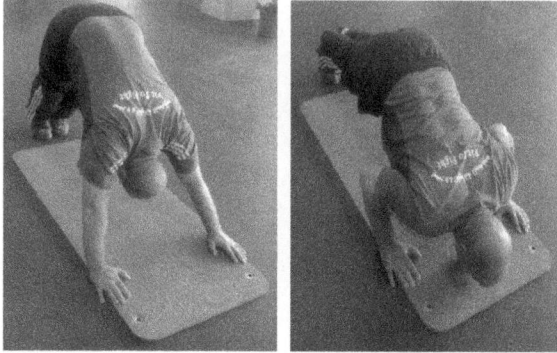

EXERCISE DESCRIPTION

With your toes on the floor, your hands level on the floor and around shoulder width apart, hold your body in a V position as best you can with your backside raised up slightly. Throughout all 3 movements your abdominals should be initiated and as you breathe out you should roll your bodyweight forwards using only your shoulders, roll down and forwards bending your arms at the elbows until your chest almost brushes the ground and then roll upwards straightening your arms and hold. Breathe in until you reverse the movement by rolling your shoulders in the opposite direction until you are back in the start position. Repeat the movement but keep the shoulders pulled down and backwards as much as possible which will ensure that your upper spine and head are relaxed and not under too much tension.

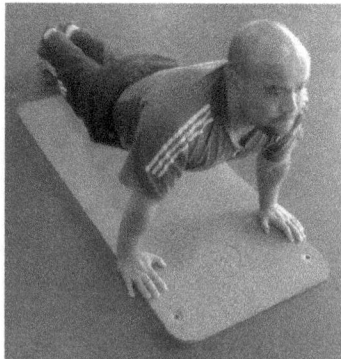

Exercise 3.5 – Additional Isometric Holds

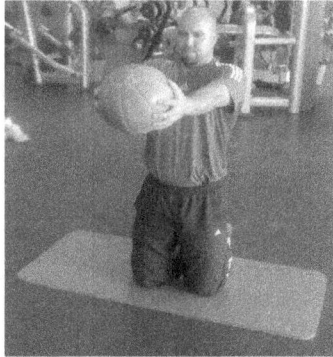

EXERCISE DESCRIPTION

Select a low enough resistance to start with until you have mastered the technique and position yourself in the kneeling or standing position. Whichever hold you are attempting your shoulders should be relaxed with your breathing as per normal. Initially you should breathe out, engage your abdominals and raise the weight up, out to the side or in front of you and hold for as long as you can throughout the different ranges of motion whilst maintaining good posture. When you feel your posture and good form faltering, control your breathing throughout but most importantly (in) as you return to the start position and repeat.

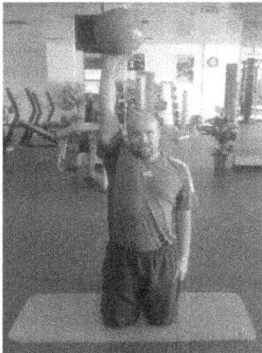

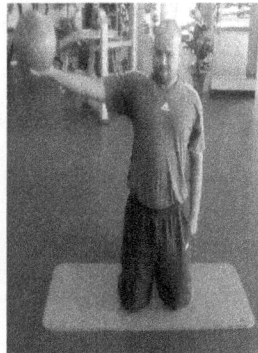

Biceps

Exercise 4.1 – Isometric hold

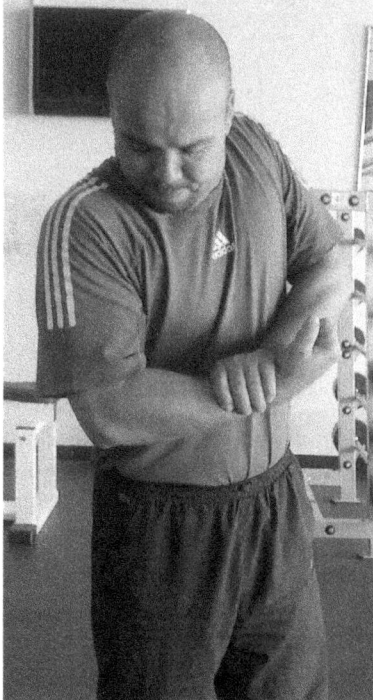

EXERCISE DESCRIPTION

Bend one of your elbows at any range and hold the wrist with your other hand, apply a resistance and attempt to fully bend your arm whilst applying a greater force. Try resisting throughout all of the ranges, hold and repeat.

Exercise 4.2 – Partner Resisted Holds

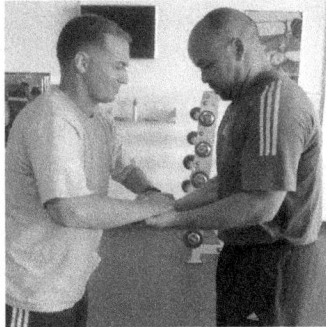

EXERCISE DESCRIPTION

Bend one or both of your elbows at any range whilst your partner holds your arm(s) ensure he/she applies a resistance as you attempt to fully bend your arm(s) as your partner applies a greater force. Try resisting throughout all of the ranges; hold and repeat (attempt both methods, left & right pictures).

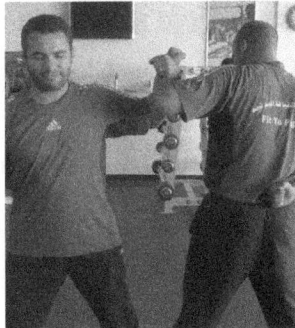

Exercise 4.3 – Under-grasp pull ups

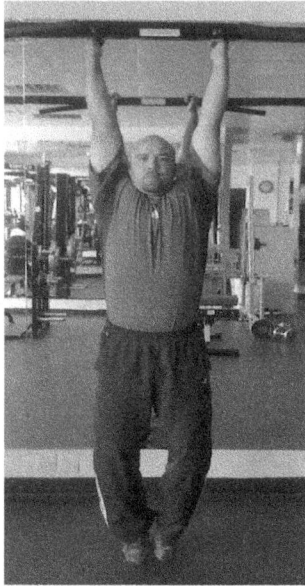

EXERCISE DESCRIPTION

Allow your body to hang in a straight line (under grasp) as you ensure that you have a tight grip on the pull up bar. Initiate your abdominals as you breathe out, pull your bodyweight up and attempt to get your chin above your hands whilst bending your arms only. Hold the position for 2-3 seconds, breathe in, lower your body under control and repeat.

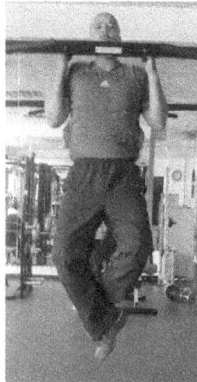

Exercise 4.4 – Behind the neck pull ups

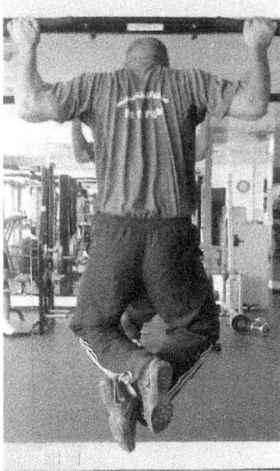

EXERCISE DESCRIPTION

Allow your body to hang in a straight line (wide grip) as you ensure that you have a tight grip on the pull up bar. Initiate your abdominals as you breathe out, pull your bodyweight up and attempt to get the back of your neck level with your hands whilst bending your arms only. Hold the position for 2-3 seconds, breathe in, lower your body under control and repeat.

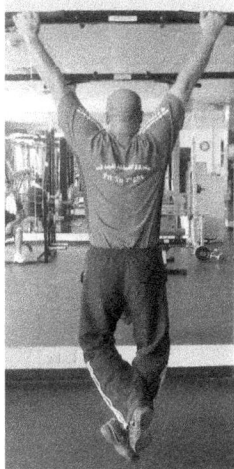

Triceps

Exercise 5.1 – Bench Dips

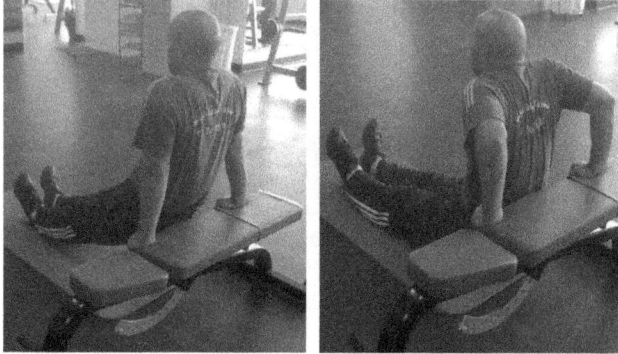

EXERCISE DESCRIPTION

Find any object that is stable, safe and secure where you can bend your elbows fully behind your body. Your aim is to place your hands firmly behind you on the bench and fairly close together. Start off with your arms straight before bending at the elbow as you breathe in, then as you breathe out raise your body upwards whilst contracting your triceps by straightening your arms. You can use the bench as above or place a chair/raised platform behind you and complete the same exercise, repeat the movement. Elevate your feet to make it more difficult.

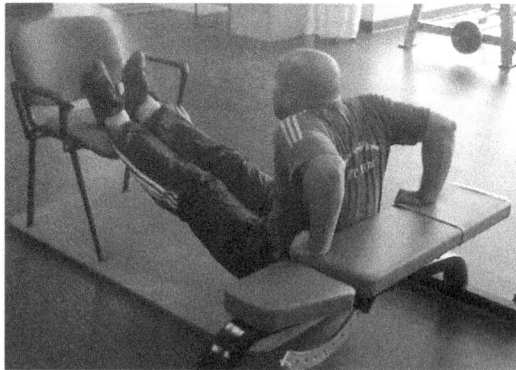

Exercise 5.2 – Incline press ups

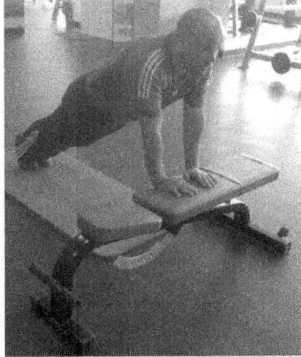

EXERCISE DESCRIPTION

Lean onto a bench/stable object ensuring that your back is straight and your shoulders relaxed whilst your hips and shoulders remain facing towards the ground along with your head and eyes. Place your hands close together before you initiate the movement from the abdominals and lower your upper body until your chest is close to the bench/stable object whilst breathing in. Breathe out as you raise your upper body back to the start position. Maintaining control throughout the movement is important whilst breathing correctly. It is very important to keep your elbows as close to the body as possible.

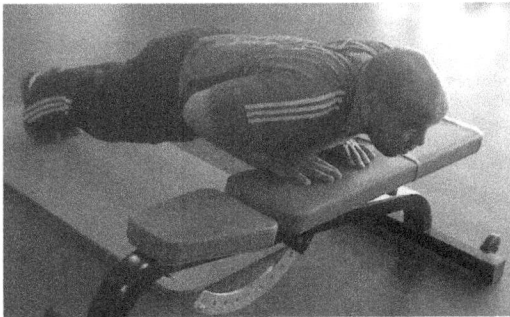

Exercise 5.3 – Advanced press ups

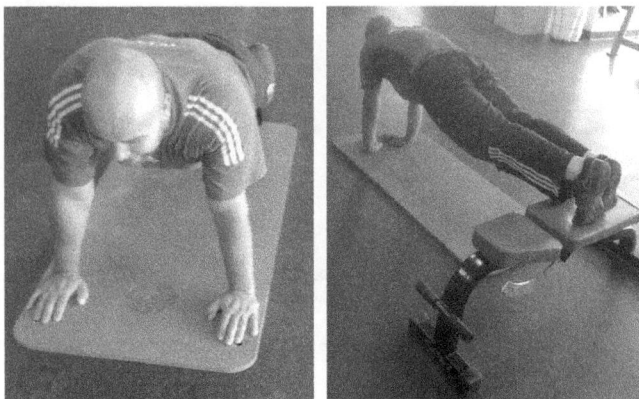

EXERCISE DESCRIPTION

With your feet on a stable raised object ensure your hands are initially level with your shoulders and your knees and hands are in line. Your shoulders should be relaxed and your hips and shoulders should remain facing towards the ground along with your head and eyes. Progress until your hands are as close together as possible before you initiate the movement from the abdominals and lower your upper body until your chest is close to the floor whilst breathing in. Breathe out as you raise your upper body back to the start position. Maintaining control throughout the movement is important whilst breathing correctly. It is very important to keep your elbows as close to the body as possible. Progress further by elevating the legs on a stable platform or unstable platform such as the fit-ball.

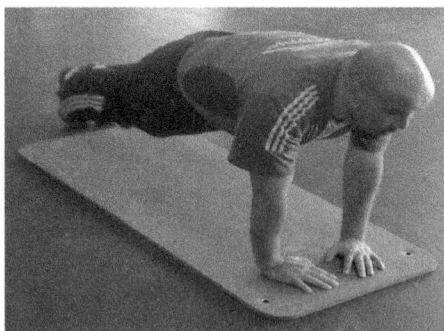

Exercise 5.4 – Partner walk

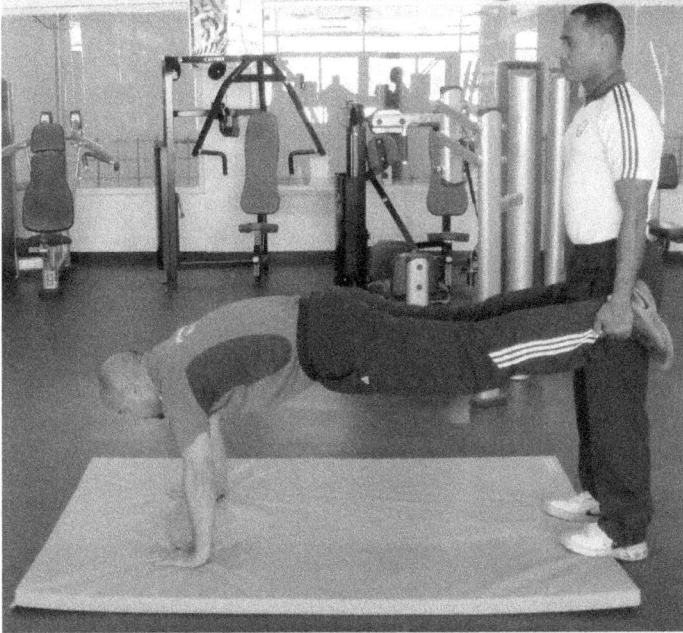

EXERCISE DESCRIPTION

Get in the press up position as your partner takes a good grip of your legs, simply walk forwards in a straight line by using your hands only. Before walking, initiate the abdominals and endeavour to keep your back straight along with the head, eyes hips and shoulders. Relax your shoulders as much as possible.

Exercise 5.5 – Body raises

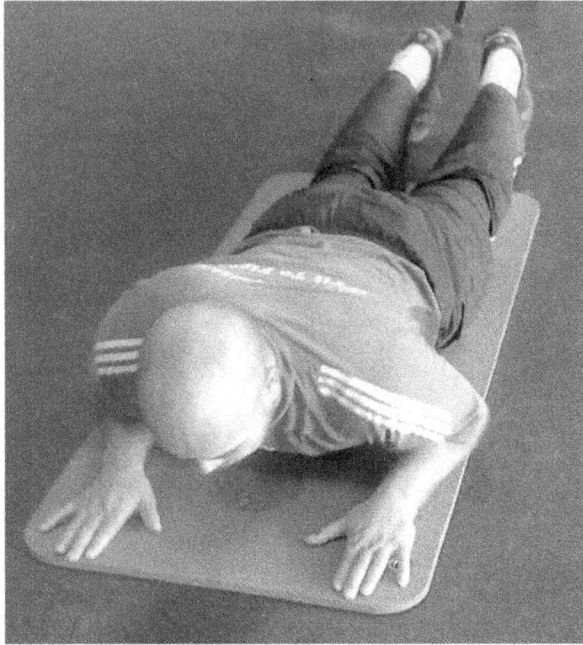

EXERCISE DESCRIPTION

Start in the front lying position with your hands level with your head shoulder width apart and with your elbows close to the sides of your body. Whilst using the arms only, initiate the abdominals and breathe out as you straighten your arms. Endeavour to keep your shoulders down and relaxed as much as possible.

Legs

Exercise 6.1 – Static Hold

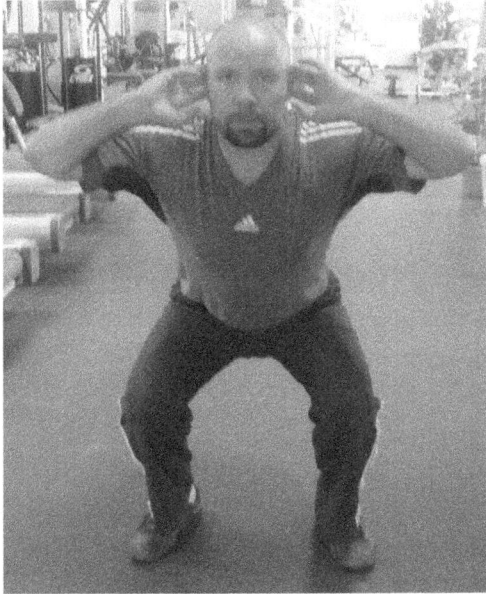

EXERCISE DESCRIPTION

Ensure that you stand with your feet flat on the floor and wide enough to maintain good balance, (normally shoulder width apart) your thighs should be parallel to the ground. Ensure your hips, shoulders, head and eyes are inline. Squat down and backwards until your knees are level with your toes. Hold the position for as long as you can, whilst breathing in a controlled manner.

Exercise 6.2 – Bridge

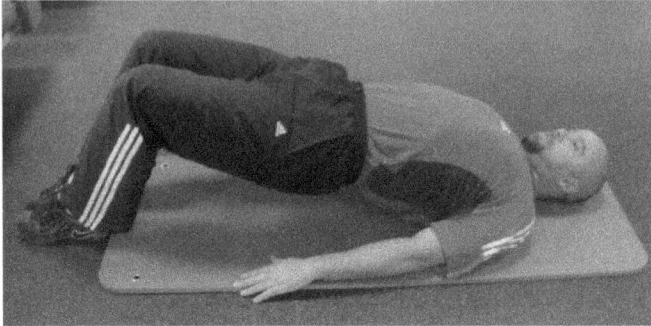

EXERCISE DESCRIPTION

In the back lying position place your feet shoulder width apart and flat on the floor with your arms relaxed by your side. Your hips, shoulders, head and eyes should be inline prior to raising your hips off the ground whilst breathing out. Breathe in as you return to the start position. Concentrate on maintaining a good body position as you raise your hips high. Use the upper leg muscles to hold you in the position. Repeat the movement in a controlled manner.

Exercise 6.3 – Squat

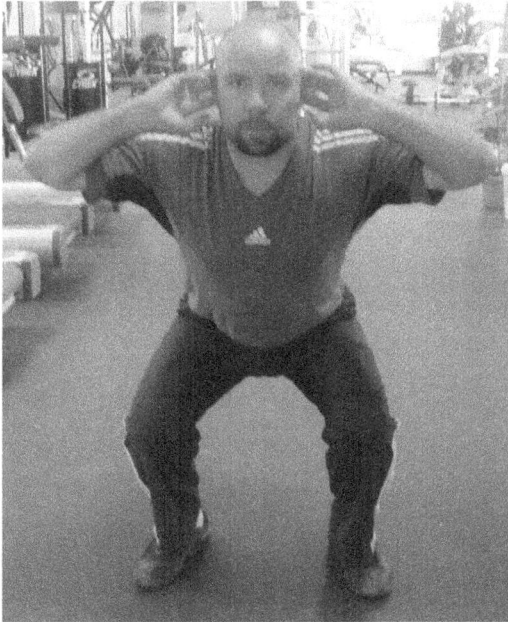

EXERCISE DESCRIPTION

Stand with your feet flat on the floor and wide enough to maintain good balance. Your hips, shoulders, head and eyes should be inline as you squat down keeping your back straight, squat down and backwards until your thighs are parallel to the ground. Ensure your knees don't go too far beyond your toes as you hold the position for 2-3 seconds before returning to the start position. Breathe in a controlled manner.

Exercise 6.4 – Lunge

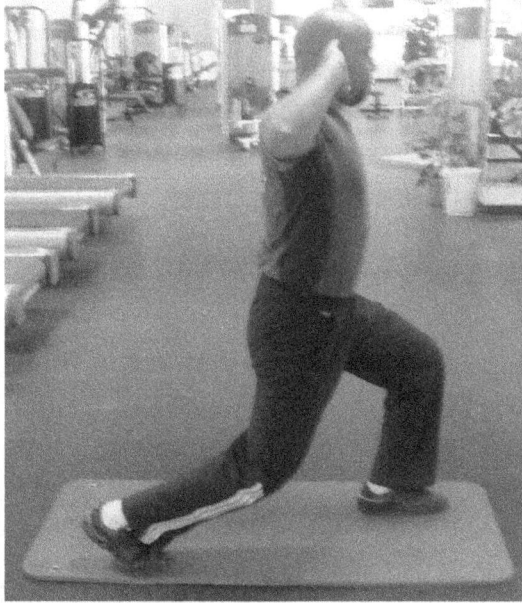

EXERCISE DESCRIPTION

Stand with your feet flat on the floor and wide enough to maintain good balance. Step backwards with one leg until the thigh of the forward leg is parallel to the ground, your hips, shoulders, head and eyes should be inline and facing forwards. Initiate the movement via the abdominals whilst keeping the back straight and breathing out, breathe in as you return to the start position and repeat. All movements should be under control and safe!! This exercise can be changed so that you step forwards instead.

Exercise 6.5 – Step Up

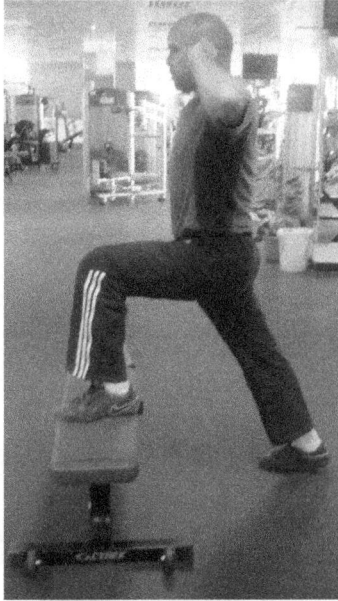

EXERCISE DESCRIPTION

Stand with your feet flat on the floor and wide enough to maintain good balance. Choose a surface that is not too low or too high and your foot is flat on it before you step up. Your hips, shoulders, head and eyes should be inline and facing forwards. Initiate the movement via the abdominals and breathe out when you step up and attempt to stand upright. As always it is very important that your back remains straight at all times. Breathe in as you return to the start position and repeat. All movements should be under control and safe!!

Exercise 6.6 – Squat Jump

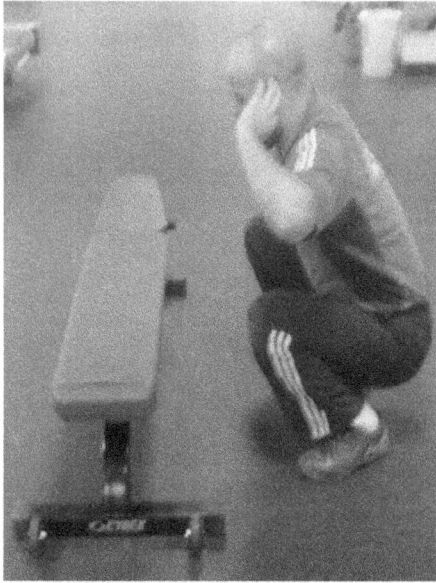

EXERCISE DESCRIPTION

Choose a stable surface to use for this exercise and start off with it up against a wall. Stand with your feet flat on the floor and wide enough to maintain good balance. Your hips, shoulders, head and eyes should be inline as you squat down keeping your back straight, squat down and backwards until your thighs are close to the ground. Breathe out as you jump forward and upwards onto the stable surface. Progress in a safe manner onto a low surface first and gradually increase the height as you become more confident. Initiating the abdominals, keeping the back straight and your breathing are very important factors whilst attempting this exercise.

Full bodyweight program – (6 week fitness base template)

Back exercises	10-30 Reps	1-6 Sets	Remarks (1-2mins rest between sets)
Back extensions			
Alt arm/leg raise 1&2			
Straight leg hold			
Plank progressions			
Hip raises			
Chest exercises	**Reps**	**Sets**	**Remarks**
Isometric hold			
Incline Push Ups			
Normal Push Ups			
Decline Push Ups			
Bodyweight Dips			
Shoulder exercises	**Reps**	**Sets**	**Remarks**
Isometric holds 1-4			
Advanced Hold			
Partner Resisted Ex's			
Caterpillar			
Additional Holds			
Bicep exercises	**Reps**	**Sets**	**Remarks**
Isometric hold			
Partner Res Holds			
Under-grasp pull ups			
Behind neck pull ups			
Triceps exercises	**Reps**	**Sets**	**Remarks**
Bench Dips			
Incline Press Ups			
Advanced press ups			
Partner walk			
Body raises			
Leg exercises	**Reps**	**Sets**	**Remarks**
Static Hold			
Bridge			
Squat			
Lunge			
Step Up			
Squat Jump			

Progress according to your fitness level
Gradually increase your effort until you have mastered perfect form and technique of all exercises i.e. from x1 set of 10 reps etc. Your intensity will be dictated by how much rest you have in between exercises and sets. You can increase the intensity by having less rest and by performing more exercises from the same muscle group i.e. overloading instead of alternating them.

CARDIOVASCULAR EXERCISE TEMPLATES

Outdoor walking – (template)

Week	Times per week	Choose the time or distance option	
		Time option (minutes)	Distance option (kilometers)
1	3	25	2.5
2	3	25	2.5
3	3	25	2.5
4	3	25	2.5
5	3	30	3.0
6	3	30	3.0
7	3	30	3.0
8	3	30	3.0
9	3	35	3.5
10	3	35	3.5
11	3	35	3.5
12	3	35	3.5
13	3	40	4.0
14	3	40	4.0
15	3	40	4.0
16	3	40	4.0

Treadmill walking – (template)

Week	Times per week	Time goal (minutes)	Speed (km/hr)	Alternate (flat / incline)	
				Flat	5%
1	3	20	5.5	-	
2	3	20	5.5	-	
3	3	20	5.5	5 mins	3 mins
4	3	20	5.5	5 mins	5 mins
5	3	25	5.5	-	
6	3	25	6.0	5 mins	5 mins
7	3	25	6.0	-	
8	3	25	6.0	-	
9	3	30	6.0	-	
10	3	30	6.0	5 mins	3 mins
11	3	30	6.5	-	
12	3	30	6.5	-	
13	3	35	6.5	-	
14	3	35	6.5	-	
15	3	35	6.5	5 mins	3 mins
16	3	35	6.5	5 mins	5 mins

Whether or not you are an experienced walker, feel free to increase or decrease the time/speed/incline guides according to your current fitness level.

Outdoor running – (template)

Week	Times per week	Activity	Choose the time or distance option	
			Time option (minutes)	Distance option (kilometers)
1	3	Walk/Run	20	2.5
2	3	Walk/Run	20	2.5
3	3	Walk/Run	20	2.5
4	3	Run	20	2.5
5	3	Run	20	2.5
6	3	Run	20	3.0
7	3	Run	20	3.0
8	3	Walk/Run	25	3.5
9	3	Walk/Run	25	3.5
10	3	Run	25	3.5
11	3	Run	25	3.5
12	3	Run	25	3.5
13	3	Run	25	4.0
14	3	Run	25	4.0
15	3	Run	25	4.0
16	3	Run	25	4.0

Treadmill running – (template)

Week	Times per week	Time goal (minutes)	Alternate			
			Walking		Running	
			Minutes	Speed (km/hr)	Minutes	Speed (km/hr)
1	3	20	3	6.8	2	11
2	3	20	2	6.8	3	11
3	3	20	2	6.8	5	11
4	3	20	2	6.8	5	11
5	3	20	-	-	20	11
6	3	25	2	6.8	5	11
7	3	25	2	6.8	5	11
8	3	25	-	-	25	11
9	3	30	2	6.8	5	11
10	3	30	2	6.8	5	11
11	3	30	-	-	30	11
12	3	30	-	-	30	11
13	3	35	2	6.8	5	11
14	3	35	2	6.8	5	11
15	3	35	-	-	35	11
16	3	35	-	-	35	11

Whether or not you are an experienced runner, feel free to increase or decrease the time/speed guides according to your current fitness level.

Outdoor cycling – (template)

Week	Times per week	Choose the time or distance option	
		Time option (minutes)	Distance option (kilometers)
1	3	20	6
2	3	20	6
3	3	20	6
4	3	20	6
5	3	25	8
6	3	25	8
7	3	25	8
8	3	25	8
9	3	30	10
10	3	30	10
11	3	30	10
12	3	30	10
13	3	35	12
14	3	35	12
15	4	35	12
16	4	35	12

Indoor cycling – (template)

Week	Times per week	Time goal in minutes	Cycling speed (rotations per minute)	Resistance
1	3	20	50+	Low
2	3	20	50+	Low
3	3	20	60+	Low
4	3	20	60+	Low/Medium
5	3	25	60+	Low/Medium
6	3	25	60+	Low/Medium
7	3	25	70+	Low/Medium
8	3	25	70+	Medium
9	3	30	70+	Medium
10	3	30	70+	Medium
11	3	30	80+	Medium
12	3	30	80+	Medium/Hard
13	3	35	80+	Medium/Hard
14	3	35	80+	Medium/Hard
15	3	35	80+	Medium/Hard
16	3	35	80+	Medium/Hard

Whether or not you are an experienced cyclist, feel free to increase or decrease the time/speed/resistance guides according to your current fitness level.

Indoor rowing – (template)

Day	Workout	Heart rate range	Total time	Average pace	Total distance (m)
Monday		-	:	:	
Tuesday		-	:	:	
Wednesday		-	:	:	
Thursday		-	:	:	
Friday		-	:	:	
Saturday		-	:	:	
Sunday		-	:	:	

Weekly combined time/distance

	:	

Stair climbing – (template)

Week	Times per week	Time goal in minutes	Exercise intensity
1	3	10	Low
2	3	10	Low
3	3	15	Low
4	3	15	Low/Medium
5	3	20	Low/Medium
6	3	20	Low/Medium
7	3	20	Low/Medium
8	3	20	Medium
9	3	25	Medium
10	3	25	Medium
11	3	25	Medium
12	3	25	Medium/Hard
13	3	30	Medium/Hard
14	3	30	Medium/Hard
15	4	30	Medium/Hard
16	4	30	Medium/Hard

Feel free to increase or decrease the time/intensity guides according to your current fitness level.

If you are exercising for long periods of time to try to burn fat why not try, "high intensity interval training" (HIIT)

How Does This Burn more fat than just Jogging?

Your metabolism goes haywire after your HIIT training session with tons of calories being burned. So essentially you burn most of the fat after your training session with HIIT training.

How Do you Perform HIIT?

Go fast… then go slow… & repeat. *Rest meaning active recovery not stopping.

You can perform HIIT routines on pretty much any cardio machine you want like an elliptical machine, a treadmill, a bike, or apply it to a sport that you enjoy like (swimming, cycling, running). Your results will be better if you can keep the bursts of speed (fast phases) at around 90%-100% of maximum effort.

Here are 2 samples of what a HIIT routine could look like:

Pre Session	Phase 1	Phase 2	Intensity	Post Session
Adequate warm up & Stretch	Sprint 20 Seconds	Rest 10 Seconds	Repeat 4-8 Times	Adequate cool down & Stretch

Pre Session	Phase 1	Phase 2	Intensity	Post Session
Adequate warm up & Stretch	Sprint 15 Seconds	Rest 5 Seconds	Repeat 4-6 Times	Adequate cool down & Stretch

Progress as you see fit i.e. 1m sprint / 3m rest or 1m sprint / 2m rest etc

You may change the routine however you choose and if you don't want to use time you can use distance i.e. as an example use lampposts which are generally evenly spaced out and sprint from one to the next and jog for 2 but remember to use fast bursts of work. The amount of times that you repeat the cycle will ultimately increase your results and increase your body's fat burning capability. Always use a workout diary so you can record your sprint timings and/or distance and of course how you felt as you repeated and increased the amount of cycles you achieved. As always, take your time, master the technique, maintain good posture throughout and try not to rush things…it will come.

All of these exercises, workout programs and more up-to-date specialist content can be found in our other books **"Exercise Your Whole Body at Home" & "Maximise your fitness potential"…** Just visit www.amazon.com or www.wholebodyworkshop.com

REFERENCES

Section 1
Willis, Judith. Drug Bulletin. Food & Drug Administration, 1996.

Section 2
Ello-Martin, Julia A., Jenny H. Ledikwe and Barbara J. Rolls. "The Influence of Food Portion Size and Energy Density on Energy Intake: Implications for Weight Management." American Journal of Clinical Nutrition 82 (2005): 236S-241S.

Calle, E. E. "Body Mass Index and Mortality." New England Journal of Medicine (1998)

Section 3
Robert E. Thayer, PhD, professor of psychology at California State University at Long Beach, "The Origin of Everyday Moods." (London: Oxford University Press, 1996).

Gavin Fitzsimons (Duke University), Joseph C. Nunes (University of Southern California), and Patti Williams (University of Pennsylvania). "License to Sin: The Liberating Role of Reporting Expectations," Journal of Consumer Research: June 2007.

Geller J, Cockell SJ, Hewitt PL, Goldner EM, Flett GL, Department of Psychiatry, University of British Columbia, Vancouver, British Columbia. Int J Eat Disord. 2000 Jul;28(1):8-19.

Diane Carlson Jones, University of Washington, Thorbjorg Helga Vigfusdottir, Reykjavik University, Yoonsun Lee, University of Washington. "Body dissatisfaction and psychological factors, Journal of Developmental Psychology, 2004.

Paxton, S. J., Neumark-Sztainer, D, Hannan, P. J, Eisenberg, M. (2006). Body dissatisfaction prospectively predicts depressive symptoms and low self-esteem in adolescent girls and boys. Journal of Clinical Child and Adolescent Psychology, 35, 539-549.

Rational Emotive Behaviour Therapy (REBT). behaviour therapies of a cognitive nature, Albert Ellis, 1953.

Section 4
Nicola Reavley, author of The Encyclopedia of Vitamins, Minerals, Supplements & Herbs, how good is the average diet? 1998 13–17

Packer, Lester, and Carol Colman. The Antioxidant Miracle. New York City: John Wiley & Sons, Inc., 1999. 185-196.

Challem, Jack. The Food-Mood Solution: All-Natural Ways to Banish Anxiety, Depression, Anger, Stress, Overeating, and Alcohol and Drug Problems – And Feel Good Again. Hoboken, New Jersey: John Riley & Sons, Inc., 2007.

Christopher Guerriero, author of Maximise Your Metabolism www.maximiseyourmetabolism.com, Unleash your metabolism, proper elimination begins with a thorough cleansing, 2005, 28-33

Van Straten, Michael. Super Energy Detox. Whitecap Books, 2003. 73.

Koh-Banerjee, Pauline, Mary Franz, Laura Sampson, Simin Liu, David R. Jacobs, Donna Spiegelman, Walter Willett, Eric Rimm. "Changes in Whole-Grain, Bran, and Cereal Fibre Consumption in Relation to 8-y Weight Gain Among Men" The American Journal of Clinical Nutrition 80 (2004): 1237-1245.

Segal-Isaacson, C.J. "First Major Study Examining Long-Term Followers of Low carbohydrate Diets." Division of Health, Behaviour and Nutrition. 2004.

Volek, J.S., M.J., Sharman, D.M. Love, N.G. Avery, A.L. Gómez, T.P. Scheet and W.J. Kraemer. "Body Composition and Hormonal Responses to a Carbohydrate-Restricted Diet." Metabolism 51 (2002): 864-870.

Ludwig, David, director. Optimal Weight for Life (OWL). Children's Hospital Boston. 10 Mar. 2008

Skov, A.R., S. Toubro, B. Ronn, L. Holm and A. Astrup. "Randomized Trial On Protein VS. Carbohydrate in Ad Libitum Fat Reduced Diet For The Treatment of Obesity." International Journal of Obesity 23 (1999): 528-536.

Johnston, Carol S. "Strategies for Healthy Weight Loss: From Vitamin C to the Glycemic Response." Journal of the American College of Nutrition 24 (2005) 158-165.

Saris, W.H., A. Astrup and A.M. Prentice. "Randomized Controlled Trial of Changes in Dietary Carbohydrate/Fat Ratio and Simple VS. Complex Carbohydrates on Bodyweight and Blood Lipids: the CARMEN Study, the Carbohydrate Ratio Management in European National Diets. International Journal of Obesity 24 (2000): 1310-1318.

Schneeman, Barbara. "Whole Grains & Health" U.S Food & Drug Administration. 2005.

Thom, Susan. "Nutrition Facts to Help Consumers Eat Smart - Food Label Changes, Focus on Food Labeling" U.S. Food & Drug Administration. May 1993.

Garcia, OZ. The Balance. New York City: ReganBooks, 1998. 113-132.

Section 5
Van Straten, Michael. Super Radiance Detox. Quadrille Publishing Ltd., 2002. 70-72.

Astrup, A., G.K. Grunwald, E.L. Melanson, W.H.M. Saris and J.O. Hill. "The Role of Low-Fat Diets in Bodyweight Control: A Meta-analysis of Ad Libitum Dietary Intervention Studies." International Journal of Obesity 24 (2000): 1545-1552.

Section 6
Jakicic, J.M. R.R. Wing, B.A. Butler and R.J. Robertson. "Prescribing Exercise in Multiple Short Bouts Versus One Continuous Bout: Effects on Adherence, Cardiorespiratory Fitness, and Weight Loss in Overweight Women." International Journal of Obesity and Related Metabolic Disorders 19 (1995), 893-901.

Stiegler, Petra and Adam Cunliffe. "The Role of Diet and Exercise for the Maintenance of Fat-Free Mass and Resting Metabolic Rate During Weight Loss." Sports Medicine 36 (2006), 239-262.

McCullagh, P, PhD. Stiehl, J. & Weiss, W.R. "Developmental modeling effects on the quantitative and qualitative aspects of motor performance." (1990).

Hill, J.O., D.G. Schlundt, T. Sbrocco, T. Sharp, J. Pope-Cordle, B. Stetson, M. Kaler and C. Heim. "Evaluation of an Alternating-Calorie Diet With and Without Exercise in the Treatment of Obesity." The American Journal of Clinical Nutrition 50 (1989). 248-254.

Section 8
Liao, K. Lih-Mei. "Cognitive-Behavioural Approaches and Weight Management: an Overview." The Journal of the Royal Society for the Promotion of Health 120 (2000): 27-30.

Section 9
Van Straten, Michael. Super Energy Detox Quadrille Publishing Ltd., 2002. 54-58

Useful websites:

www.resolutions.bz
www.nhlbi.nih.gov
www.weight-dieting.org
www.bestdietforme.com
www.web4health.info
www.wikipedia.com
www.lifestylewtloss.com/
www.athealth.com/Consumer/disorders/Bingeeating.html
www.weightlosspsychology.com
www.dashdiet.org

INDEX

www.ingramcontent.com/pod-product-compliance
Lightning Source LLC
Chambersburg PA
CBHW030010290326
41934CB00005B/285